OMEGA 3 FATTY ACIDS

OMEGA 3 FATTY ACIDS

ROBERT P. HARRIS

Novinka Books
An imprint of Nova Science Publishers, Inc.
New York

NOTICE TO THE READER

The Publisher has taken reasonable care in the preparation of this book, but makes no expressed or implied warranty of any kind and assumes no responsibility for any errors or omissions. No liability is assumed for incidental or consequential damages in connection with or arising out of information contained in this book. The Publisher shall not be liable for any special, consequential, or exemplary damages resulting, in whole or in part, from the readers' use of, or reliance upon, this material.

This publication is designed to provide accurate and authoritative information with regard to the subject matter covered herein. It is sold with the clear understanding that the Publisher is not engaged in rendering legal or any other professional services. If legal or any other expert assistance is required, the services of a competent person should be sought. FROM A DECLARATION OF PARTICIPANTS JOINTLY ADOPTED BY A COMMITTEE OF THE AMERICAN BAR ASSOCIATION AND A COMMITTEE OF PUBLISHERS.

Library of Congress Cataloging-in-Publication Data:
Available upon request

ISBN 1-59454-690-8

Published by Nova Science Publishers, Inc. ✢ New York

CONTENTS

PREFACE

The Food and Drug Administration (FDA) announced the availability of a qualified health claim for reduced risk of coronary heart disease (CHD) on conventional foods that contain eicosapentaenoic acid (EPA) and docosahexaenoic acid (DHA) omega-3 fatty acids.

Typically, EPA and DHA omega-3 fatty acids are contained in oily fish, such as salmon, lake trout, tuna and herring. These fatty acids are not essential to the diet; however, scientific evidence indicates that these fatty acids may be beneficial in reducing CHD.

"Coronary heart disease is a significant health problem that causes 500,000 deaths annually in the United States," said Dr. Lester M. Crawford, Acting FDA Commissioner. "This new qualified health claim for omega-3 fatty acids should help consumers as they work to improve their health by identifying foods that contain these important compounds."

A qualified health claim on a conventional food must be supported by credible scientific evidence. Based on a systematic evaluation of the available scientific data, as outlined in FDA's "Interim Procedures for Qualified Health Claims in the Labeling of Conventional Human Food and Human Dietary Supplements", FDA is announcing a qualified health claim for EPA and DHA omega-3 fatty acids. While this research is not conclusive, the FDA intends to exercise its enforcement discretion with respect to the following qualified health claim:

"Supportive but not conclusive research shows that consumption of EPA and DHA omega-3 fatty acids may reduce the risk of coronary heart disease. One serving of [name of food] provides [x] grams of EPA and DHA omega-3 fatty acids. [See nutrition information for total fat, saturated fat and cholesterol content.]

In 2000, the FDA announced a similar qualified health claim for dietary supplements containing EPA and DHA omega-3 fatty acids and the reduced risk of CHD. FDA recommends that consumers not exceed more than a total of 3 grams per day of EPA and DHA omega-3 fatty acids, with no more than 2 grams per day from a dietary supplement.

The EPA and DHA omega-3 fatty acid qualified health claim is only the second qualified health claim that FDA has announced for conventional food.

Chapter 1

QUESTIONS AND ANSWERS

QUALIFIED HEALTH CLAIM FOR OMEGA-3 FATTY ACIDS, EICOSAPENTAENOIC ACID (EPA) AND DOCOSAHEXAENOIC ACID (DHA)

1. What action has FDA taken today?
2. What is the difference between a qualified health claim and an unqualified health claim?
3. What products can use the qualified health claim?
4. Are omega-3 fatty acids essential to a healthy diet?
5. What foods contain omega-3 fatty acids?
6. What are the benefits of omega-3 fatty acids?
7. How much omega-3 fatty acids should I consume in my diet?
8. What happens if I consume more the recommend amounts of omega-3 fatty acids?
9. Since FDA is announcing this claim, does this mean that FDA has scientific evidence that consumption of omega-3 fatty acids reduces the risk of coronary heart disease?
10. FDA has warned consumers about tuna and mercury. Doesn't this qualified health claim contradict this warning?
11. Can all fish use this qualified health claim?
12. Since fresh fish is not labeled, how will consumer know which fish have these fatty acids?

Q: What action has FDA taken today?
A: FDA announced a qualified health claim for the use of eicosapentaenoic acid (EPA) and docosahexaenoic acid (DHA) omega-3 fatty acids for conventional foods and dietary supplements.

Q: What is the difference between a qualified health claim and an unqualified health claim?
A: Both types of health claims characterize a relationship between a substance (specific food component or a specific food) and a disease or health-related condition, and are supported by scientific evidence. All health claims must undergo review by FDA through a petition process. All unqualified health claims must meet the Significant Scientific Agreement standard as provided for by Congress in 1990. Court decisions resulting in qualified health claims focused on a manufacturer's right to make statements about diet/disease relationships when the science supporting the claim did not meet the Significant Scientific Agreement standard, provided that the claim about the relationship was stated or "qualified" in such a way as to not mislead consumers. Thus, qualified health claims differ from unqualified ones in the level of scientific support and in that they must be accompanied by a disclaimer or otherwise qualified.

Q: What products can use the qualified health claim?
A: FDA will consider its enforcement discretion, effective immediately, for food products labeled with the qualified health claim. Food products labeled with the qualified health claim must contain both EPA and DHA omega-3 fatty acids.

Q: Are omega-3 fatty acids essential to a healthy diet?
A: Alpha-linolenic acid is the only essential omega-3 fatty acid and is found in vegetable oil, e.g. flax seed. EPA and DHA omega-3 fatty acids are synthesized in the body and are not essential although there is supportive but not conclusive research to show that these fatty acids are beneficial in reducing the risk of coronary heart disease.

Q: What foods contain omega-3 fatty acids?
A: Foods that contain omega-3 fatty acids include fatty fish such as salmon, lake trout, tuna, and herring.

Q: What are the benefits of omega-3 fatty acids?

A: Supportive but not conclusive research has shown that EPA and DHA omega-3 fatty acids may reduce the risk of coronary heart disease.

Q: How much omega-3 fatty acids should I consume in my diet?

A: FDA recommends that consumers not exceed more than a total of 3 grams per day, with no more than 2 grams per day from a dietary supplement.

Q: What happens if I consume more the recommend amounts of omega-3 fatty acids?

A: Some scientific studies show that consumption levels well over 3 grams per day may lead to excessive bleeding. Therefore, FDA recommends that consumption not exceed 3 grams per day from all food sources.

Q: Since FDA is announcing this claim, does this mean that FDA has scientific evidence that consumption of omega-3 fatty acids reduces the risk of coronary heart disease?

A: FDA has determined that there is supportive, but not conclusive, scientific evidence that suggests a reduction in coronary heart disease as a result of eating foods rich in omega-3 fatty acids. This important health benefit will help consumers as they work to improve their diets by selecting foods that will benefit their health.

Q: FDA has warned consumers about tuna and mercury. Doesn't this qualified health claim contradict this warning?

A: FDA's fish advisory is directed to a specific population--women of childbearing age, pregnant women, nursing mothers and young children. This qualified health claim does not contradict the advisory; instead it makes consumers aware of the benefits of consuming fish. The advisory addresses the issue of the types and amounts of fish to consume for the specific subpopulation (women of childbearing age, pregnant women, nursing mothers and young children) to reduce their exposures to the harmful effects of mercury.

Q: Can all fish use this qualified health claim?

A: FDA will consider its enforcement discretion for the use of the qualified claim for fish that contain EPA and DHA omega-3 fatty acids such as salmon, lake trout, tuna, and herring.

Q: Since fresh fish is not labeled, how will consumers know which fish have these fatty acids?

A: As part of the qualified health claim language, products that bear the qualified health claim will say how much EPA and DHA omega-3 fatty acid will be present in a serving.

If a product bears a qualified health claim, consumers may find information on the amount of EPA and DHA omega-3 fatty acid on labels affixed to the food or through other labeling including shelf labels, signs, posters, brochures that are readily available and in close proximity to the fish.

Chapter 2

FDA LETTERS RELATED TO OMEGA-3 FATTY ACIDS AND REDUCED RISK OF CORONARY HEART DISEASE

LETTER RESPONDING TO HEALTH CLAIM PETITION DATED JUNE 23, 2003 (WELLNESS PETITION): OMEGA-3 FATTY ACIDS AND REDUCED RISK OF CORONARY HEART DISEASE (DOCKET NO. 2003Q-0401)

Jonathan W. Emord, Esq.
Emord & Associates, P.C.
1800 Alexander Bell Drive, Suite 200
Reston, VA 20191

RE: Health Claim Petition: Omega-3 Fatty Acids and Reduced Risk of Coronary Heart Disease (Docket No. 2003Q-0401)

Dear Mr. Emord:

This letter responds to the health claim petition dated June 23, 2003, submitted to the Food and Drug Administration (FDA or the agency), on behalf of Wellness Lifestyles, Inc. and Life Extension Foundation Buyers Club (collectively, Wellness petition) pursuant to Sections 403(r)(4) and 403 (r)(5)(D) of the Federal Food, Drug, and Cosmetic Act (the Act) (21 U.S.C.

§§ 343(r)(4) and 343(r)(5)(D)). The petition requested that the agency authorize a health claim characterizing the relationship between the consumption of omega-3 fatty acids (specifically, eicosapentaenoic acid (EPA) and docosahexaenoic acid (DHA)) and a reduced risk of coronary heart disease (CHD). The petition requested that the disclaimer on the existing omega-3 fatty acids and CHD dietary supplement health claim, as stated in a letter dated October 31, 2000[1] (subsequently modified by a letter dated February 16, 2001[2] and by a letter dated February 8, 2002[3]) be removed and that the claim be extended to omega-3 fatty acid containing foods. This petition proposed the model health claim: "Consumption of omega-3 fatty acids may reduce the risk of coronary heart disease."

FDA evaluated the scientific evidence provided with the petition and other evidence related to your claim. Based on this review, FDA determined that the scientific evidence supporting the proposed health claim does not meet the "significant scientific agreement" standard under 21 U.S.C. § 343 (r)(3)(B)(i) of the Act. FDA notified you of this decision and you submitted a letter on August 12, 2003 agreeing to the petition being reviewed as a qualified health claim. Thus, FDA filed the petition on September 3, 2003 as a qualified health claim petition and posted it on the FDA website for a 60-day comment period, consistent with the agency's guidance for procedures on qualified health claims.[4]

FDA received a qualified health claim petition (the Martek petition) from Mr. Martin J. Hahn on November 4, 2003, as both a petition and a comment on your petition. Mr. Hahn submitted the petition on behalf of Martek Biosciences Corporation. The Martek petition requested an extension of the existing omega-3 fatty acid and CHD dietary supplement qualified health claim to conventional foods, including foods fortified with omega-3 fatty acids (specifically EPA and DHA). Because the substance and disease and the request for an extension of the existing omega-3 fatty acids and CHD qualified health claim were the same in each petition, FDA consolidated the petitions in the same docket (Docket No. 2003Q-0401).

The agency received several comments on the petitions. You submitted two comments. Other comments were from industry, a professional organization, and an individual. The comments addressed various issues including the substance of the claim, mercury content in fish, minimum effective levels of EPA and DHA, disqualifying nutrient levels, minimum nutrient content requirements, and claim statements. All support extending the omega-3 fatty acid qualified health claim to conventional foods. FDA considered the relevant comments in its evaluation of this petition.

This letter sets forth the basis of FDA's determination that the current evidence for the proposed health claim is appropriate for consideration for a qualified health claim on conventional foods and dietary supplements. This letter also sets out the factors that FDA intends to consider for the exercise of its enforcement discretion for a qualified health claim, for both conventional foods and dietary supplements, with respect to consumption of EPA and DHA omega-3 fatty acids and a reduced risk of coronary heart disease. This letter is an update to the previous letters on the use of a qualified health claim on EPA and DHA omega-3 fatty acid dietary supplements and coronary heart disease risk (the October 31, 2000 letter,[5] the February 16, 2001 letter,[6] and the February 8, 2002 letter[7]) and provides FDA's current thinking with respect to the use of this qualified health claim on both dietary supplements and conventional foods. Throughout the text of this letter, the phrase "omega-3 fatty acid qualified health claim" will be used to refer to the qualified health claim about the consumption of EPA and DHA omega-3 fatty acids and a reduced risk of coronary heart disease.

I. Overview of Data and Eligibility for a Qualified Health Claim

In a review of a qualified health claim, FDA considers the data and information provided in the petition, in addition to other data and information available to the agency that may assist in its review of the relationship between the substance and the disease or health-related condition. Consistent with its guidance entitled "Interim Evidence-based Ranking System for Scientific Data,"[8] the agency evaluates the scientific studies to determine what studies are pertinent to its review in evaluating the relationship. The agency may conclude that certain design flaws in a study are so significant that the study may not be helpful to the agency's decision about whether the particular study supports a relationship. Such design flaws may include the lack of a control group or the lack of any analysis of the data (Spilker et al., 1991; Federal Judicial Center, 2000).

In addition to human studies, FDA also considers other data and information in its review, such as meta-analyses[9], review articles[10], and animal[11] and in vitro[12] studies. These other types of data and information are useful in assisting the agency with an understanding of the scientific issues about a disease or health-related condition, but generally do not themselves establish a health claim relationship in the absence of supporting human intervention or observational data.

After the agency decides what scientific studies are relevant to its review about whether there is evidence to support a relationship between a substance and a disease or health-related condition, (i.e., what studies to rate based on study quality), the agency categorizes these studies into: (1) the most persuasive studies, which are studies designed to evaluate whether there is a relationship between the substance and disease outcome (e.g., intervention studies that manipulate the intake level of the substance while controlling for other factors that can affect disease risk reduction and/or; (2) less persuasive studies (e.g., studies that my have design flaws that make them less reliable in evaluating a substance/disease relationship or less applicable to the U.S. population (conducted in countries where usual intakes of the substance is much lower or higher than in the U.S.). The most persuasive studies are given the greatest consideration. FDA rates the most and less persuasive studies for quality. Scientific quality is based on several criteria including study population, intervention design (e.g., presence of a placebo control), data collection (e.g., dietary assessment method), statistical analysis, and outcome measures. For example, if the scientific study adequately addressed all or most of the above criteria, it would receive a high quality rating. Lower quality ratings (e.g., moderate and low) would be given based on the extent of the deficiencies or uncertainties in the quality criteria.

Collectively, FDA then rates the strength of the total body of evidence that it determines is relevant to its review, using criteria such as the study type (e.g., intervention), quality, quantity (number of the various types of studies and sample sizes), and consistency of the results. Based on the totality of the scientific evidence, FDA determines whether such evidence is credible to support the substance/disease relationship, and if so, then determines the ranking that reflects the level of comfort among qualified scientists that such a relationship is scientifically valid.

The Wellness petition cited 24 publications as evidence to substantiate the relationship for this claim. These publications consisted of 6 reports of intervention studies,[13] 8 observational studies,[14] 3 review articles,[15] 1 position paper from the American Heart Association,[16] 1 editorial,[17] 1 meta-analysis of intervention studies on omega-3 and CHD,[18] 1 food composition survey,[19] and 3 in vitro studies.[20]

The agency did not consider all the publications cited in the Wellness petition to be pertinent to its review of this substance/disease relationship. While useful for background information, the review articles, position paper and meta-analysis did not contain sufficient information on the individual studies reviewed and therefore FDA could not determine their pertinence regarding factors such as the study population characteristics or the composition of the products used (e.g., food, dietary supplement); similarly, the lack of detailed information on the studies summarized in the review articles, position paper and meta-analysis did not allow FDA to determine if the studies are flawed in critical elements such as its design, execution, and data analysis. FDA must review the scientific quality of a study to determine whether credible conclusions can be drawn from it. The food composition survey measured how much omega-3 fatty acid was in a given food. FDA did not consider the food composition survey as pertinent because it did not measure whether omega-3 fatty acids reduced the incidence of disease or affected a surrogate endpoint for CHD. FDA did not consider the in vitro studies that were submitted in the petition as providing any supportive information about the substance/disease relationship because in vitro models of disease are conducted in artificial environments that cannot mimic normal physiology that may be involved in the risk reduction of CHD, nor can in vitro models mimic the human body's response to consumption of omega-3 fatty acids.

In addition to the studies in your petition that the agency considered, FDA considered 7 intervention studies (5 from the Martek petition[21]; 1 from a comment[22]; 1 identified by FDA through a literature search[23]), 3 observational studies from the Martek petition[24]and 2 chapters from a report compiled by the Institute of Medicine from the Martek petition.[25]

A. Substance

A health claim characterizes the relationship between a substance and a disease or health-related condition (21 CFR 101.14(a)(1)). A substance means a specific food or component of food (21 CFR 101.14(a)(2)). The petitions identified the omega-3 fatty acids, eicosapentaenoic acid (EPA) and docosahexaenoic acid (DHA), as the substance for the proposed claim. EPA and DHA are components of some fatty fish (primarily cold water fish),[26] fish oils, other foods (e.g., seaweed), dietary supplements, and food ingredients (e.g., algal oils). Therefore, the agency concludes that the substances, EPA and DHA omega-3 fatty acids, identified in the petition are components of food and therefore meet the definition of substance in the health claim regulation (21 CFR 101.14(a)(2)).

B. Disease or Health-Related Condition

A disease or health-related condition means damage to an organ, part, structure, or system of the body such that it does not function properly, or a state of health leading to such dysfunctioning (21 CFR 101.14(a)(5)). The petition has identified coronary heart disease (CHD) as the disease for the proposed claim. The agency concludes that CHD is a disease and therefore that the petitioner has satisfied the requirement in 21 CFR 101.14(a)(5).

C. Safety Review

Under 21 CFR 101.14(b)(3)(ii), if the substance is to be consumed at other than decreased dietary levels, the substance must be a food or a food ingredient or a component of a food ingredient whose use at levels necessary to justify a claim must be demonstrated by the proponent of the claim, to FDA's satisfaction, to be safe and lawful under applicable food safety provisions of the Federal Food, Drug, and Cosmetic Act.

The Wellness petition stated that omega-3 fatty acids, as EPA and DHA, have been a naturally occurring ingredient in foods consumed safely in the United States prior to January 1, 1958, and that there is no evidence that when consumed either in foods or as dietary supplements there is a cumulative effect in the diet that is unsafe. The Martek petition stated that omega-3 fatty acids occur in conventional foods with a long history of safe use, such as fish, and are generally recognized as safe (GRAS) when used as direct food ingredients intended to increase omega-3 fatty acids. Some comments to the petition expressed an interest in using the omega-3 fatty acid qualified health claim for foods that contain EPA and DHA as a food ingredient from sources including fish oil and algal oil.

In order to meet the safe and lawful requirement for health claims (21 CFR 101.14(b)(3)(ii)), the use of EPA and DHA omega-3 fatty acids, when used in conventional food or as a dietary supplement at levels necessary to justify the claim, must be demonstrated, to FDA's satisfaction, to be safe and lawful. FDA evaluates whether the substance is "safe and lawful" under the applicable food safety provisions of the Act. For conventional foods, this evaluation involves considering whether the ingredient that is the source of the substance is GRAS, approved as a food additive, or authorized by a prior sanction issued by FDA (see 21 CFR 101.70(f)). Dietary ingredients in dietary supplements, however, are not subject to the food additive provisions of the act (see section 201(s)(6) of the Act (21 U.S.C. § 321(s)(6)). Rather, they are subject to the adulteration provisions in section 402 of the Act (21 U.S.C. 342) and, if applicable, the new dietary ingredient provisions in section 413 of the Act (21 U.S.C. 350b), which pertain to dietary ingredients that were not marketed in the United States before October 15, 1994. The term "dietary ingredient" is defined in section 201(ff)(1) of the act and includes vitamins; minerals; herbs and other botanicals; dietary substances for use by man to supplement the diet by increasing the total daily intake;

and concentrates, metabolites, constituents, extracts, and combinations of the preceding types of ingredients.

In 1997, FDA affirmed, as GRAS, menhaden oil as a direct human food ingredient with specific limitations of use to ensure that the total daily intake of EPA and DHA would not exceed 3.0 grams per person per day (g/p/d) (62 FR 30751; June 5, 1997; 21 CFR184.1472). EPA and DHA are the major omega-3 fatty acids in fish oil and together comprise about 20 percent by weight of menhaden oil. FDA established maximum use levels of menhaden oil in certain foods because of concerns over possible adverse effects of fish oil consumption on bleeding time, glycemic control, and LDL cholesterol (62 FR 30751 at 30757; June 5, 1997). In 2002, FDA published a proposed rule to reallocate the uses of menhaden oil in conventional food, while maintaining the total daily intake of EPA and DHA from menhaden oil at a level not exceeding 3.0 g/p/d (67 FR 8744; February 26, 2002). FDA placed specific limitations, including the category of foods, the functional use of the ingredient, and the level of use, to ensure that the consumption of EPA and DHA from conventional food sources would not exceed 3.0 g/p/d. FDA then published a tentative final rule (69 FR 2313; January 15, 2004) to additionally require that menhaden oil not be used as an ingredient in foods in combination with other added oil that is a significant source of EPA and DHA to ensure that total intake from conventional food sources do not exceed 3.0 g/p/d.

In addition, FDA has not objected to certain GRAS notifications for additional sources of EPA and DHA as food ingredients (fish oils other than menhaden oil) (GRAS Notice Nos: GRN000097, GRN000102, GRN000105, GRN000109, GRN 000137, GRN000138).[27] These GRAS notices proposed maximum use levels consistent with those specified in the tentative final rule affirming, as GRAS, menhaden oil as a direct human food ingredient with specific limitations of use.

FDA has also responded without objection to a GRAS notification on algal oil DHA from Martek Biosciences Corporation. Martek estimated that the use of algal oil in a number of food categories at the maximum proposed use levels would result in a mean exposure of no more than 1.5 grams of DHA per day (GRAS Notice No. GRN000137).

The mean exposure to EPA and DHA from menhaden oil in all conventional food categories is estimated to be 2.7 g/p/d (67 FR 8744 at 8746; February 26, 2002). This is a conservative estimate with substantial margin for safety, and the agency believes, consistent with its prior decision on the use of a qualified health claim for DHA and EPA omega-3 fatty acids (October 31, 2000 letter), that the addition of menhaden oil to food products has not come close to this conservative mean estimate exposure. FDA further believes that the GRAS uses for which it received a GRAS notification for other sources of EPA and DHA omega-3 fatty acids also provide conservative estimates of exposure and that the addition of these EPA and DHA sources to food products do not come close to the conservative mean estimates. Not all foods in the marketplace within those permitted food categories would contain menhaden oil or other sources of EPA and DHA omega-3 fatty acids that substitute for other edible fat or oil. Also, because not all foods that a consumer eats every day would contain menhaden or other EPA and DHA oil used as a substitute oil, the actual total daily intakes of EPA and DHA from menhaden or other EPA and DHA oil for an average person should be significantly below 3.0 g/p/d (67 FR 8744 at 8746; February 26, 2002).

It is difficult to estimate the actual total consumption of EPA and DHA. The Continuing Survey of Food Intakes by Individuals (1994-1996, 1998)[28] estimated EPA and DHA intakes from conventional foods.[29] The 50th percentile intake of EPA and DHA from the survey was between 0.06 g and 0.07 g for adult women and 0.07 g and 0.1 g for adult men. The 90th percentile intake was between 0.18 g and 0.22 g for women and between 0.20 g and 0.43 g for men. Thus, EPA and DHA consumption from conventional foods in the United States is low. FDA is not aware of any nationally representative consumption data on EPA and DHA from dietary supplements. In the October 31, 2000 letter, FDA expressed concern about the exposure to EPA and DHA omega-3 fatty acids potentially exceeding 3.0 g/p/d if a qualified health claim were to appear on dietary supplements. This concern was due to conventional foods containing omega-3 fatty acids that were on the market; the use of structure/function claims on products containing EPA and DHA omega-3 fatty acids, which may promote product purchase; and dietary supplements that FDA found in the marketplace that contained significant amounts of EPA and DHA.

With this letter, the requested use of this qualified health claim is now extended to conventional foods. The agency believes that there is likely to be some increased consumption of EPA and DHA omega-3 fatty acids based on conventional foods that bear the qualified health claim; however, the amounts of EPA and DHA that can be used and the foods in which such food ingredients can be safely used are limited. The agency has established specific limitations of use under its menhaden oil GRAS rule (62 FR 30751; June 5, 1997), proposed and tentatively finalized reallocation of the use of menhaden oil without changing total exposure levels (67 FR 8744; February 26, 2002, 69 FR 2313; January 15, 2004). Also, manufacturers that have submitted GRAS notifications for other sources, to which the agency has not objected, have established conditions of use similar to those in the menhaden oil GRAS rule.

In the October 31, 2000 letter,[30] FDA stated that a consumer could consume nearly 1 gram of EPA and DHA per day in the diet from conventional foods. The agency is uncertain about how much consumers will increase their intake of EPA and DHA omega-3 fatty acids from EPA and DHA containing conventional foods and dietary supplements due to the extended use of the qualified health claim. In order to help consumers gauge their total intake of EPA and DHA and to provide them a way to keep their intake of EPA and DHA within 3 grams per day, FDA intends to consider, as a factor in the exercise of its enforcement discretion, that conventional foods and dietary supplements that bear an omega-3 fatty acid qualified health claim declare the amount of EPA and DHA per serving in the claim. FDA recommends that the information on EPA and DHA content for use in a qualified health claim for EPA and DHA omega-3 fatty acids and reduced risk of CHD be presented in a manner that is consistent with FDA's guidance entitled, "FDA Nutrition Labeling Manual--A Guide for Developing and Using Data Bases." You may contact CFSAN's Office of Nutritional Products, Labeling, and Dietary Supplements (ONPLDS) for further information. The dietary supplement may declare the amount of EPA and DHA per serving in "Supplement Facts," instead of making the declaration in the claim. Also, to ensure further that consumers do not exceed a 3.0 g/p/d intake, FDA will educate consumers not to exceed 3.0 g/p/d from all food and dietary supplement sources through print and web outreach information. Further, FDA intends to consider, as a factor in the exercise of its enforcement discretion, that dietary supplements not recommend or suggest in labeling that consumers ingest more than 2 grams of EPA and DHA per day. FDA encourages manufacturers to limit their dietary supplement products bearing the qualified health claim to products recommending or suggesting daily intake of 1 gram or less of EPA and DHA omega-3 fatty acids.

Based on the data and information that FDA considered, which includes data and information that FDA relied upon in reaching its conclusions about the safety of EPA and DHA omega-3 fatty acids in its GRAS affirmation of menhaden oil, the data and information in the 1991 proposed (56 FR 60663; November 27, 1991) and 1993 final rules (58 FR 2683; January 6, 1993), and its current scientific literature review for other possible safety concerns, FDA concludes that the use of EPA and DHA omega-3 fatty acids used as a GRAS ingredient, consistent with FDA's GRAS rule for menhaden oil and

GRAS notifications to which FDA did not object, and the use as a dietary supplement is safe and lawful under 21 CFR 101.14 provided that daily intakes of EPA and DHA omega-3 fatty acids from conventional food and dietary supplement sources do not exceed 3.0 g/p/d. In section IV, FDA sets forth factors under which it plans to exercise enforcement discretion for EPA and DHA containing conventional foods and dietary supplements bearing the qualified claim, to ensure, among other things, that such use will be safe.

II. The Agency's Consideration of a Qualified Health Claim

FDA has identified the following endpoints to use in identifying CHD risk reduction for purposes of a health claim evaluation for EPA and DHA omega-3 fatty acids: Coronary events (MI, ischemia), cardiovascular death, atherosclerosis, and high blood pressure. Artherosclerosis is the underlying cause of CHD, which can lead to the signs of CHD including coronary events (MI, ischemia) and cardiovascular death.[31] High blood pressure, serum total cholesterol, serum LDL-cholesterol, and serum HDL-cholesterol are considered as surrogate endpoints for CHD.[31] However, FDA concluded in its October 31, 2000 letter[32] that omega-3 fatty acids do not affect serum cholesterol levels (total, LDL, HDL). To evaluate the potential effects of EPA and DHA omega-3 fatty acid consumption on CHD risk, FDA considered coronary events (myocardial infarction (MI), ischemia), cardiovascular death, atherosclerosis, and high blood pressure as indicators or predictors of disease.

In considering the qualified health claim for EPA and DHA omega-3 fatty acid dietary supplements in October 2000, FDA focused on human data that had become available since FDA's 1991-93 review and on human studies that quantitatively measured or estimated the omega-3 fatty acid intakes in relation to a direct measure of CHD risk or a surrogate endpoint for CHD risk. Several, but not all, of the studies[33] that FDA had considered in its October 31, 2000 letter were submitted in these current petitions. Studies that have been published since that letter were also included in the petitions. For purposes of this review, FDA, in determining the scientific support for a relationship between EPA and DHA omega-3 fatty acid dietary supplements and CHD, focused on the more recent studies to determine whether these studies added any support to the scientific evidence that was used for the current qualified health claim for EPA and DHA omega-3 fatty acid dietary supplements. For purposes of determining whether there is a relationship between EPA and DHA omega-3 fatty acids from conventional foods and reduced risk of CHD, FDA determined whether the relevant studies cited in the petition, in addition to other relevant studies that the agency had already reviewed in its previous reviews, support a qualified health claim.

A. Assessment of the Intervention Studies

FDA identified a total of 10 intervention studies, not previously reviewed in 2000, for its current review of this qualified health claim (3 from the current petition[34]; 5 from the Martek petition [35]; 1 from a comment[36]; 1 identified by FDA through a literature search[37]). FDA did not consider some of these studies in its current review for the following reasons: 1) Marchioli, et al. (2002) was a reanalysis of GISSI et al. (1999), which FDA reviewed in 2000, and provided no additional evidence relevant for establishing a substance-disease relationship; 2) Thies et al. (2003) and Maresta et al. (2002) measured outcomes (plaque stability and percutaneous transluminal coronary angioplasty (PTCA), respectively) that are not recognized as valid surrogate endpoints for CHD; 3) the studies by Ghafoorunissa et al. (2002), Laidlaw and Holub, et al. (2003) did not include control groups for EPA and DHA (Spilker, 1991); 4) Leng et al. (1998) did not include a control for gamma-linolenic acid (GLA), which constituted the majority of the treatment (approximately six times higher than EPA), thus there is no way to determine whether the effects were due to EPA; and 5) two intervention studies that reported no benefit on CHD incidence (Angerer et al., 2002; Nilsen et al., 2001) were conducted in CHD patients and the results could not be extrapolated to the general healthy population; therefore, these data were not considered relevant to FDA's review for establishing a substance-disease relationship in the general population. Thus, FDA considered only 2 intervention studies identified since the 2000 review as capable of supporting the substance/disease relationship (Finnegan et al., 2003; Woodman et al., 2002).

The studies by Finnegan et al. (2003) and Woodman et al. (2002) were randomized, placebo-controlled, double-blind[38] intervention studies that reported the effects of fish oil on blood pressure. Finnegan et al. (2003) reported the results from a study involving 150 moderately hyperlipidemic subjects[39] assigned to 1 of 5 interventions: fish oil (0.8 or 1.7 g/day EPA+DHA); rapeseed and linseed oil (4.5 or 9.5 g/day ALA), or an n-6 PUFA control (sunflower and safflower oil) for 6 months. The fish oil intervention provided no benefit in CHD risk factors, including blood pressure, compared to the placebo control group. Woodman et al. (2002) was a 6-week intervention comparing EPA ethyl ester[40] (4 g/day) or DHA ethyl ester40 (4 g/day) with olive oil (4 g/day) in type 2 diabetics[41] with hypertension (n=52). Neither EPA ethyl ester nor DHA ethyl ester provided any benefit to blood pressure or any other CHD risk factor compared with the olive oil treated patients.

B. Assessment of the Observational Studies

FDA identified 10 observational studies not previously reviewed in 2000. These consisted of 6 prospective cohort studies (4 from the current petition[42]; 2 from the Wellness petition[43]), 3 nested case-control studies from the current petition,[44] and 1 ecological study from the Martek petition.[45]

Two of the 10 studies on fish consumption and CHD[46] were not considered in this review because these studies only reported total fish consumption without providing details of the fish type[47] or portion sizes, thus there is no way of knowing how much, if any, EPA and DHA omega-3 fatty acid was consumed. The remaining 8 observational studies[48] were of high to moderate quality. These observational studies provide only an estimated intake of EPA and DHA omega-3 fatty acids from fish consumption and provided only an association with disease risk, and not direct causality of disease risk.

Hu et al. (2002) reported results from the Nurses' Health Study, a prospective cohort study on female registered nurses (n=84,688) with a 16 year follow-up. Fish and omega-3 fatty acid intake were calculated as an average intake from all available dietary questionnaires up to the start of each 2-year follow-up interval in which events were reported. There was an inverse correlation observed between fish/omega-3 fatty acid consumption and incidence of CHD, including CHD deaths and nonfatal MI. A subgroup analysis of diabetic nurses from this cohort (n=5,103; Hu et al., 2003) observed a reduced risk of CHD from fish consumption but the association did not extend to estimated EPA and DHA omega-3 fatty acid consumption.

Albert et al. (2002) was a case-control study nested in the U.S. Physicians Health Study (Albert et al., 1998), which was considered in the 2000 review. The nested case-control study had a 17-year follow-up and reported a significant inverse relationship between whole blood omega-3 fatty acid concentrations and CHD death.

The study by Rissanen et al. (2000) reported 10-year follow-up results from the Kuopio Ischemic Heart Disease Risk Factor Study, which is an ongoing, prospective, population-based cohort study investigating risk factors for cardiovascular disease (CVD) and is part of the World Health Organization's (WHOs) MONICA project. The study enrolled 1,871 men who had no clinical CHD at baseline examination. The authors reported a decrease in acute coronary events in men at the highest quintile[49] of serum DHA+DPA[50] concentration compared with men at the lowest quintile.

Results from the Cardiovascular Health Study were reported by Mozaffarian et al. (2003). In this prospective cohort study, men (~1,500) and women (~2,400) aged >65 years were enrolled who were free of known CVD at baseline in 1989-1990 and had data on fish consumption. During the 9.3 years of follow-up, there were 247 ischemic heart disease (IHD)[51] deaths and 363 MIs. Estimated intake of EPA + DHA at baseline (0.55 g/day and 0.92 g/day) was associated with lower risk of fatal ischemic heart disease (IHD), but there was no association between EPA + DHA and non-fatal MI. This result is consistent with the report from a case-control study nested in the Cardiovascular Health Study (Lamaitre et al., 2003). A higher plasma concentration of EPA + DHA was associated with a lower risk of fatal IHD, but there was no association between plasma concentration of EPA + DHA and a risk of non-fatal IHD.

Hallgren et al. (2001) was a case-control study nested in the Västerbotten Intervention Programme, which was part of the WHOs MONICA project. In this study, 78 people (cases) developed an MI, and were matched against 156 controls subjects that were randomly selected from the study. Fish intake was assessed by a food frequency questionnaire (FFQ).[52] In addition, fatty acid composition of the plasma phospholipids, including EPA and DHA, was analyzed. There was no correlation between fish intake or blood EPA+DHA and acute MI.

Torres et al. (2000) compared fish consumption in Portuguese men living in a fishing village (n=50) or rural village (n=37) with IHD-related deaths based on death certificate records for the population. There was significantly more fish consumed in the fishing village compared with the rural village and this correlated with lower IHD deaths estimated from death certificate records for the two villages.

C. Other Data and Information

The Institute of Medicine (IOM) of the National Academy of Sciences has stated in its most recent Macronutrient Report that "Growing evidence suggests that dietary n-3 polyunsaturated fatty acids (eicosapentaenoic acid [EPA] and docosahexaenoic acid [DHA]) reduce the risk of coronary heart disease (CHD) and stroke."[53] Therefore, by concluding that there was only "growing evidence" that is "suggestive" of the relationship for this proposed claim, the IOM recognized limitations in the current data on omega-3 and its ability to reduce risk of CHD.

III. Strength of the Scientific Evidence

FDA relies primarily on human studies that are primary reports of data collection when attempting to establish a diet-disease relationship and has consistently identified two endpoints with which to identify disease risk reduction for purposes of health claims evaluations: a) reduction in incidence of the disease, and; b) beneficial changes in surrogate endpoints for the disease.[54] The most persuasive evidence for a relationship between EPA and DHA omega-3 fatty acids and reduced risk of CHD would be from intervention studies with EPA and DHA omega-3 fatty acids demonstrating reduced incidence of CHD in healthy populations (i.e., primary prevention). However, no such studies for EPA and DHA omega-3 fatty acids and CHD were identified. There were 2 small intervention studies in healthy populations that measured EPA and DHA effects on blood pressure, a CHD surrogate endpoint, but no benefit was observed in these studies. Thus, the scientific evidence from intervention studies available since the 2000 review with EPA and DHA omega-3 fatty acids as the test substance, did not show a relationship between omega-3 fatty acids and reduced risk of CHD in the general population.

The remaining studies considered were high to moderate quality observational studies on healthy populations. Of these, 3 studies (Albert et al., 1998, 2002; Hu et al., 2002; Mozaffarian et al., 2003 (also Lamaitre et al., 2003)) were conducted in populations relevant to the general U.S. population, across a broad age range (30 to 84 years) and consistently reported that EPA and DHA omega-3 fatty acids reduced the risk of CHD. The largest cohorts followed 84,688 women (Hu et al., 2002) and 20,551 men (Albert et al., 1998, 2002). Of the observational studies conducted in populations considered less relevant to the general U.S. population, 1 small study (n=78 cases) (Hallgren et al. 2001) reported no benefit; whereas 2 studies (Rissanan et al, 2000; Torres et al., 2000) with sample sizes of 1,871 and 50, respectively, reported an associated benefit. Observational studies provide less compelling evidence than intervention studies for a relationship between omega-3 fatty acids and reduced risk of CHD because they provide only an estimated intake of EPA and DHA omega-3 fatty acids rather than a direct measure. In addition, observational studies cannot separate the effect of EPA and DHA omega-3 fatty acids from the effects of other food components, and therefore it is not clear whether any purported benefit is related to the EPA and DHA omega-3 fatty acids or to other dietary factors. Observational studies provide only supportive rather than direct evidence for a relationship. For these reasons, FDA considers observational studies as less persuasive than intervention studies conducted in a general healthy population for establishing a substance-disease relationship. Nevertheless, primary prevention of CHD in healthy populations by EPA and DHA omega-3 fatty acids was observed in the majority of observational studies reviewed, which included 2 large prospective cohorts conducted in the US, the Nurses' Health Study (n=84,688; 16 year follow-up; Hu et al., 2002) and the U.S. Physicians Health Study (n=20,551; 11 to 17 year follow-up; Albert et al., 1998, 2002). In sum, the majority of observational studies consistently observed an associated CHD risk reduction from intake of EPA and DHA estimated from the diet in men and women in populations relevant (3 studies) or less relevant (2 studies) to the general U.S. population.

Given the inability of predicting CHD risk reduction in a general healthy population based on secondary prevention studies in diseased populations, and the limitations of the observational studies in separating the effects of EPA and DHA omega-3 fatty acids from other dietary factors, the agency evaluated other available evidence, as discussed in the October 31, 2000 letter, that provide support for a qualified health claim for EPA and DHA omega-3 fatty acids and reduced risk of CHD. As described in detail in the October 31, 2000 letter,[55] FDA considered: (1) observational studies in the general healthy population in which fish consumption was the primary contributor of EPA and DHA omega-3 fatty acids, and (2) intervention studies in both the general healthy population and patients with established CHD that evaluated the effects of EPA and DHA omega-3 fatty acids on physiological endpoints (e.g., total cholesterol, LDL-cholesterol, HDL-cholesterol, VLDL-cholesterol, triglycerides, platelet aggregation), some of which have been proposed as possible mechanisms for the CHD risk reduction by EPA and DHA omega-3 fatty acids. Thus, FDA is not changing its position from that outlined in the October 31, 2000 letter on the EPA and DHA omega-3 fatty acid and CHD qualified claim that there is sufficient suggestive evidence that the benefit on CHD reported in CHD patients (i.e., secondary prevention) (reviewed in the October 31, 2000 letter) applies to the general population because of: (1) The primary CHD prevention in the general population associated with EPA and DHA consumption from fish in observational studies; and, (2) intervention studies demonstrating similar physiological effects of EPA and DHA in both the diseased and general populations. FDA still concludes that the weight of the scientific evidence for a health claim for EPA and DHA omega-3 fatty acids outweighs the scientific evidence against such a claim. The most significant change in the available body of evidence since 2000 is the additional observational studies, the majority of which consistently reported an associated benefit in CHD risk from EPA and DHA consumption from fish.

The observational studies estimating EPA and DHA omega-3 fatty acid intake from conventional foods support the expansion of the existing qualified health claim for EPA and DHA omega-3 fatty acids from dietary supplements and CHD to conventional foods. Therefore, FDA intends to consider the exercise of its enforcement discretion with regard to a qualified health claim on the label or in labeling of EPA and DHA omega-3 fatty acid-containing dietary supplements and conventional foods that provides a truthful and non-misleading description of the strength of the body of scientific evidence, e.g., "supportive but not conclusive research shows." Other factors that FDA intends to consider in deciding whether to exercise its enforcement discretion with regard to the use of this qualified health claim on particular foods, including dietary supplements, are discussed below.

IV. Other Enforcement Discretion Factors

Factors that FDA intends to consider in the exercise of its enforcement discretion for qualified health claims about EPA and DHA omega-3 fatty acids and reduced risk of coronary heart disease are discussed below. You should also know that FDA is considering its enforcement discretion as applying only to such foods in which EPA and DHA is an added ingredient that FDA has approved as a food additive or affirmed as GRAS or for which the agency has received a GRAS notification to which it did not object.

A. Total Fat, Saturated Fat, and Cholesterol Criteria for CHD-related Health Claims

In regulations authorizing CHD-related health claims, FDA has generally required, with a few exceptions, that foods bearing such claims meet the "low fat" criterion defined by 21 CFR 101.62(b)(2), the "low saturated fat" criterion defined by 21 CFR 101.62(c)(2), and the "low cholesterol" criterion defined by 21 CFR 101.62(d)(2) (see authorized claims in 21 CFR sections 101.75, 101.77, 101.81, 101.82, and 101.83). The agency discusses below how the agency intends to consider these criteria as factors in deciding whether to exercise its enforcement discretion for an omega-3 fatty acid qualified health claim on conventional foods and dietary supplements. Later in Section B, FDA discusses total fat, saturated fat, and cholesterol content disqualifying levels relative to the general requirement for health claims (21 CFR 101.14(a)(4)).

"Low Fat" Criterion

FDA has required in the past that foods bearing CHD health claims meet the requirement for "low fat" as defined by 21 CFR 101.62(b)(2). The requirement of the "low fat" criterion was first introduced in the dietary lipid and cardiovascular disease proposed rule (56 FR 60727 at 60739; November 27, 1991). FDA stated that, although total fat is not directly related to increased risk for CHD, it may have significant indirect effects. The agency stated that low fat diets facilitate reduction in the intake of saturated fat and cholesterol to recommended levels. Furthermore, the agency noted that obesity is a major risk factor for CHD, and dietary fats, which have more than twice as many calories per gram as proteins and carbohydrates, are major contributors to total calorie intakes. There have been several exceptions to this criterion in the past. Instead of the "low fat" criterion, fish and game meat are required to meet the "extra lean" criterion in the saturated fat and cholesterol and CHD health claim (21 CFR 101.75(c)(2)(ii)). Products derived from whole soybeans without added fat are exempted from the "low fat" criterion in the soy protein and CHD health claim (21 CFR 101.82(c)(2)(iii)(C)). In the plant sterol/stanol esters and CHD health claim, FDA does not require the "low fat" criterion but requires that total fat level of foods not exceed the total fat disqualifying level (21 CFR 101.14(a)(4)) with an exception for spread and dressing for salad on a per 50 g basis (21 CFR 101.83(c)(2)(iii)(C)). In not requiring the "low fat" criterion, FDA noted that the Dietary Guidelines for Americans, 2000 (USDA & DHHS, 2000) recommended choosing a diet that is low in saturated fat and cholesterol and moderate in total fat. Specifically, the Dietary Guidelines recommended moderate amounts of foods high in unsaturated fat with a caution to avoid excess calories.

FDA concurs with the dietary guidelines that consuming diets low in saturated fat and cholesterol is more important in reducing CHD risk, than consuming diets low in total fat. Therefore, FDA has decided not to consider, as a factor in the exercise of its enforcement discretion, that either dietary supplements or conventional foods that bear an omega-3 fatty acid qualified health claim meet the "low fat" criterion.

"Low Saturated Fat" and "Low Cholesterol" Criteria

In regulations authorizing CHD health claims, FDA has also generally required that foods bearing the claims meet the "low saturated fat" criterion as defined by 21 CFR 101.62(c)(2), and the "low cholesterol" criterion as defined by 21 CFR 101.62(d)(2) (see authorized claims in 21 CFR sections 101.75, 101.77, 101.81, 101.82, and 101.83). FDA continues to believe that these criteria are important. Therefore, FDA intends to consider, as a factor in the exercise of its enforcement discretion, that conventional foods or dietary supplements that bear an omega-3 fatty acid qualified health claim meet the "low saturated fat" and "low cholesterol" criteria. However, there are some situations, as discussed below, when FDA does not believe that such a factor is important to a decision about the exercise of its enforcement discretion.

Low Saturated Fat

FDA intends to consider, as a factor in the exercise of its enforcement discretion, that individual foods other than fish that bear an omega-3 fatty acid qualified health claim, meet the "low saturated fat" criterion (21 CFR 101.62(c)(2)). This food category includes primarily foods enriched with EPA- and DHA-containing food ingredients. FDA intends to consider, as a factor in the exercise of its enforcement discretion for meal products as defined in 21 CFR 101.13(l) and main dishes as defined in 21 CFR 101.13(m) that such foods meet all criteria specified for the "low saturated fat" criteria (21 CFR 101.62(c)(2)). FDA believes that many foods would meet the "low saturated fat" criteria, as stated in the final rule for nutrient content claims (58 FR 2302 at 2339; January 6, 1993). The criteria, "no more than 15 percent of calories from saturated fat" for individual foods can be achieved due to calorie contribution from food ingredients other than fish oil in these foods. Later in this section, FDA defines fish as "products that are essentially all fish" and identifies nutrient content factors that it intends to consider in the exercise of its enforcement discretion for the qualified health claim.

FDA intends to exercise its enforcement discretion for EPA- and DHA-containing dietary supplements (whether softgels or liquid forms) that bear an omega-3 fatty acid qualified health claim, and that meet the low saturated fat criterion per reference amount customarily consumed (RACC). However, FDA does not intend to consider, as a factor in the exercise of its enforcement discretion, that "no more than 15 percent of calories be from saturated fat." In a fish oil, 20 - 30 percent of calories come from saturated fat (USDA National Nutrient Database for Standard Reference, Release 17). Because 100 percent fish oil dietary supplements usually have no other source of calories other than fish oil and reformulation is not possible to reduce percent of calories from saturated fat, fish oil dietary supplements would not be eligible for the qualified health claim if FDA decided to consider the 15 percent criterion in 21 CFR 101.62(c)(2) as a factor in the exercise of its enforcement discretion. FDA believes that not considering the

15 percent criterion as a factor in the exercise of its enforcement discretion is appropriate given that fish oils are derived from fish, which have been shown to be associated with a reduced risk of CHD in observational studies with healthy individuals. In the algal oil used in Martek's dietary supplements, 40 - 45 percent of the oil is DHA and 30 - 40 percent of calories come from saturated fat.[56] Because the algal oil is diluted by high oleic sunflower oil by 7 - 10 percent or by 50 - 60 percent to make the final DHA concentration specific to Martek's products (either 20 percent or 40 percent DHA), calorie contribution from saturated fat will be either a little less than 30 - 40 percent (for the 40 percent DHA product) or about 15 - 20 percent of calories (for the 20 percent DHA product). In the final oil, calories from saturated fat exceed 15 percent; however, the level overlaps with that of fish oils. Therefore, FDA intends to consider, as a factor in the exercise of its enforcement discretion, that dietary supplements that bear an omega-3 fatty acid qualified health claim meet the "equal to or less than 1 g of saturated fat per RACC" criterion in 21 CFR 101.62(c)(2) but does not intend to consider the "no more than 15 percent of calories from saturated fat" criterion as a factor in the exercise of its enforcement discretion.

Low Cholesterol

FDA intends to exercise enforcement discretion for an omega-3 fatty acid qualified health claim for individual foods, other than fish and dietary supplements, provided that such foods meet the low cholesterol criteria (21 CFR 101.62(d)(2)). The October 31, 2000 letter[57] and subsequent letters from FDA[58], [59] did not discuss the low cholesterol criteria for dietary supplements; however, most fish oil containing dietary supplements do not meet the low cholesterol criteria per 50 g. Most dietary supplements containing EPA and DHA omega-3 fatty acids (whether fish oils or algal oils) are in softgels, and the amount of these oils per RACC is very small. Serving sizes are usually in between 1 - 2 softgels. FDA estimates that 1 - 2 softgels may weigh about 1 - 3 g, containing about 0.5 - 2 g of fish oil or algal oil. This amount of fish oil would not exceed the "low cholesterol" criteria (20 mg) per RACC but would exceed the "low cholesterol" criteria per 50 g basis if the supplements contain 100 percent fish oil. Liquid forms of fish oil dietary supplements are much less common and provide usually one teaspoon as a serving size (containing 4.5 g of total fat). This amount of fish oil may contain about 22 - 34 mg of cholesterol (based upon USDA National Nutrient Database for Standard Reference, Release 17), but again such levels of consumption would not be common.

Algal oil dietary supplements are sold as softgels and the RACC of the supplement is one softgel, containing 0.5 g of the mixture of algal oil and high oleic sunflower oil.[60] Both the 100 mg DHA softgel and the 200 mg DHA softgel contain less than 2 mg of cholesterol, which is below the "low cholesterol" criteria (20 mg) per RACC. The cholesterol content of algal oil will vary. The algal oil that Martek proposed to use for various food categories in its GRAS notification (GRAS No. 000137) contains higher levels of cholesterol (about 380 mg/100g without dilution) than does the algal oil currently used for dietary supplements (about 30 mg/100g without dilution). Even if the algal oil with the high cholesterol content were used for dietary supplements, the cholesterol content per RACC would be very small (about 2 mg of cholesterol) because the amount of oil per serving (0.5 g) is small, but the cholesterol content would exceed the "low cholesterol" criteria (20 mg) per 50 g basis.

FDA estimates that 50 g of fish oils would contain about 240 to 380 mg of cholesterol (USDA National Nutrient Database for Standard Reference, Release 17). The algal oil currently used for dietary supplements (without the addition of sunflower oil) contains about 15 mg of cholesterol per 50 g.[61] The algal oil that Martek proposed to use for foods in its GRAS notification (GRAS No. 000137) (without the addition of sunflower oil) contains about 190 mg of cholesterol per 50 g.

Since it is highly unlikely that individuals would consume 50 g of dietary supplements containing EPA and DHA per day, FDA has decided that it is not necessary to consider, as a factor in the exercise of its enforcement discretion, that EPA- and DHA-containing dietary supplements weighing equal to or less than 5 g per RACC contain no more than 20 mg of cholesterol on a 50 g basis. However, FDA has decided that it is necessary to consider, as a factor in the exercise of its enforcement discretion, that EPA- and DHA-containing dietary supplements that weigh more than 5 g per RACC contain no more than 20 mg of cholesterol on a 50 g basis.

"Extra Lean" Criterion for Fish

FDA has defined fish in 21 CFR 123.3(d) as "fresh or saltwater finfish, crustaceans, other forms of aquatic animal life (including, but not limited to, alligator, frog, aquatic turtle, jellyfish, sea cucumber, and sea urchin and the roe of such animals) other than birds or mammals, and all mollusks, where such animal life is intended for human consumption." For the purpose of omega-3 fatty acid qualified health claims about fish, FDA intends to consider certain factors in the exercise of its enforcement discretion for use of these claims on "products that are essentially all fish." This category includes fish without any added ingredients and fish with a small amount of added fat or carbohydrate that meets the definition of an insignificant amount in 21 CFR 101.9(f)(1). Examples of "products that are essentially all fish" are raw fish, boiled fish, and broiled fish.

In the past, fish was given an exception for the "low saturated fat" criterion and "the low cholesterol" criterion, along with game meat, in the health claim about diets low in saturated fat and cholesterol and reduced risk of CHD (21 CFR 101.75 (c)(2)(ii)). Instead of the "low saturated fat and low cholesterol" criteria, fish was required to meet the "extra lean" criterion as defined in 21 CFR 101.62(e)(3) (i.e, contains less than 5 g total fat, less than 2 g saturated fat, and less than 95 mg cholesterol per reference amount customarily consumed and per 100 g.).

In applying the "extra lean" criterion to fish, FDA was not thinking about oily fish that are rich in EPA and DHA omega-3 fatty acids. Most fish that are a rich source of EPA and DHA exceed the "extra lean" criterion for saturated fat (2 g of saturated fat per RACC) but do not exceed the saturated fat disqualifying level (4 g of saturated fat per RACC). One of the ways that FDA determines whether to consider nutrient content eligibility criteria as a factor in the exercise of its enforcement discretion is whether there are risk reduction data among healthy individuals that would suggest that there may be a benefit from consumption of the food, even though the food does not meet the nutrient content eligibility criteria. Such data, for purposes of this review, would include an association with a lower risk of CHD, shown in observational studies conducted in apparently healthy individuals. Because the following observational studies: Albert et al., 1998, 2002; Hu et al., 2002; Mozaffarian et al., 2003 showed an association of fish intake with reduced risk of CHD in apparently healthy individuals, FDA has decided that the agency does not need to consider, as a factor in the exercise of its enforcement discretion for products that are essentially all fish, that such products meet the "extra lean" criterion for saturated fat. However, FDA has decided to consider, as a factor in the exercise of its enforcement discretion for products that are essentially all fish, that such products meet the "extra lean" criterion for cholesterol (95 mg of cholesterol per RACC). Most fish that are rich sources of EPA and DHA do not exceed the "extra lean" criterion for cholesterol; thus, this approach should not disqualify many products that are essentially all fish. As discussed earlier, FDA now considers the "low fat" criterion not important here; therefore, FDA is not considering the "extra lean" criterion for total fat, as a factor in exercising its enforcement discretion, which is not very different from how the agency approached its consideration of the "low fat" criteria as a factor for products that are essentially all fish.

B. Disqualifying Nutrient Levels

Under the general requirements for health claims (21 CFR 101.14(e)(3)) a food may not bear a health claim if that food exceeds any of the disqualifying nutrient levels for total fat, saturated fat, cholesterol, or sodium established in § 101.14(a)(4). Section 101.14 applies to all health claims regardless of types of diseases and health-related conditions. The disqualifying nutrient levels vary for individual foods, meal products, and main dishes. Disqualifying total fat levels are above 13.0 g per RACC, per label serving size and per 50 g if the RACC is 30 g or less or 2 tablespoons or less for individual foods, above 26.0 g per label serving size for meal products, and above 19.5 g per label serving size for main dish products. Disqualifying saturated fat levels are above 4.0 g per RACC, per label serving size and per 50 g if the RACC is 30 g or less or 2 tablespoons or less for individual foods, above 8.0 g per label serving size for meal products, and above 6.0 g per label serving size for main dish products. Disqualifying cholesterol levels are above 60 mg per RACC, per label serving size and per 50 g if the RACC is 30 g or less or 2 tablespoons or less for individual foods, above 120 mg per label serving size for meal products, and above 90 mg per label serving size for main dish products. Disqualifying sodium levels are 480 mg per RACC, per label serving size and per 50 g if the RACC is 30 g or less or 2 tablespoons or less for individual foods, above 960 mg per label serving size for meal products, and above 720 mg per label serving size for main dish products.

The general requirements for health claims also provide for FDA to authorize a health claim for food despite the fact that a nutrient in the food exceeds the disqualifying level, if the agency finds that such a claim will assist consumers in maintaining healthy dietary practices. In such cases, the label must also bear a disclosure statement that complies with 21 CFR 101.13(h), highlighting the nutrient that exceeds the disqualifying level (21 CFR 101.14(e)(3)).

The application of these regulatory provisions to omega-3 fatty acid qualified health claims on dietary supplements and conventional foods is discussed below.

"Total fat" Disqualifying Level

In the previous section (Section IV A), FDA explained that the agency has decided not to consider, as a factor in the exercise of its enforcement discretion, that dietary supplements and conventional foods that bear an omega-3 fatty acid qualified health claim meet the "low fat" criterion as defined by 21 CFR 101.62(b)(2). FDA notes that there is a large difference in the amount of total fat between the "low fat" criterion and the disqualifying total fat level. For example, the "low fat" criterion for individual foods is equal to or less than 3 g per RACC and per 50 g if RACC is 30 g or less or 2 tablespoons or less. The total fat disqualifying level for individual foods is above 13 g per RACC, per label serving size and per 50 g if RACC is 30 g or less or 2 tablespoon or less. Thus, there is a difference of 10 g for individual foods between the "low fat" criterion and the total fat disqualifying level. In addition, the disqualifying levels of nutrients are a required element of all health claims (i.e., cancer claims, osteoporosis claims, CHD claims) under 21 CFR 101.14. Because FDA has not evaluated the implications of eliminating the total fat disqualifying level for all possible health claims, FDA believes that it would be appropriate to consider, as a factor in the exercise of its enforcement discretion that conventional foods and dietary supplements that bear an omega-3 fatty acid qualified claim meet the total fat disqualifying level. However, there are some situations, as discussed below, when FDA does not believe that such a factor is important to a decision about the exercise of its enforcement discretion.

Products that are Essentially All Fish

Based upon the data the agency has (USDA National Nutrient Database for Standard Reference, Release 17), FDA believes that total fat content of almost all fish that are a rich source of EPA and DHA are below the total fat disqualifying level (13.0 g of total fat per RACC). A few fish including halibut, herring, and mackerel contain total fat exceeding 13 g but contain less than 16.0 g of total fat per RACC. Because the observational studies that showed an association of fish intake with reduced risk of CHD do not distinguish fish species, FDA has no basis to discriminate one type of fish from any other type. In addition, the amount of total fat exceeding the disqualifying total fat level by these fish is small (about 3 g); therefore, FDA has decided to consider, as a factor in the exercise of its enforcement discretion, that products that are essentially all fish not exceed a total fat content per RACC of 16.0 g. If the total fat level of products that are essentially all fish exceeds the disqualifying level as defined by 21 CFR 101.14(a)(4), the disclosure statement (i.e., "See nutrition information for total fat, saturated fat, and cholesterol content") required by §101.14(e)(3) must be placed immediately adjacent to and directly beneath the claim, with no intervening material, in the same size, typeface, and contrast as the claim itself. Under 21 CFR 101.9(j)(10), if raw fish bears a health claim, nutrition labeling of the fish must be presented to the public in accordance with 21 CFR 101.45. Nutrition labeling of fish other than raw fish must follow the regulations specified in 21 CFR 101.9.

Other Conventional Foods and Dietary Supplements

Unlike fish, other EPA- and DHA-containing conventional foods that contain high levels of total fat have not been shown to have an association with a reduced risk of CHD in a population free of CHD. Therefore, FDA intends to consider the "total fat" disqualifying levels as defined in 21 CFR 101.14(a)(4) for all conventional foods, other than products that are essentially all fish, in the agency's consideration for the exercise of enforcement discretion for the omega-3 qualified health claim.

A comment suggested that FDA apply 6.5 g or less of total fat per RACC and per labeled serving instead of the "low fat" criterion as an eligibility criterion for spreads and mayonnaise-type dressings and requested an exemption for these foods from the "low fat" criterion and the total fat disqualifying level per 50 g. As explained earlier in this letter (Section IV A), FDA does not intend to consider the "low fat" criterion as a factor in the exercise of its enforcement discretion for the omega-3 qualified health claim. The 50 g weight-based criterion was developed, in part, to deal with foods with small serving sizes (e.g., foods with 15-30 g RACCs) that are dense in nutrients such as fat or sodium. As the agency noted in the final rule for general requirements for health claims, foods with small serving sizes may be consumed more frequently than once a day (58 FR 2478 at 2496; January 6, 1993). Health claims on foods such as spreads (RACC is 15 g) and mayonnaise-type dressings (RACC is 15 g) would promote their consumption, and could contribute to large intakes of total fat and calories that might not help to maintain healthy dietary practices. In addition, the level of scientific evidence linking EPA and DHA omega-3 fatty acids to reduced risk of CHD does not reach the significant scientific evidence standard; therefore, there is a fair amount of uncertainty as to whether frequent consumption of EPA and DHA enriched spreads and mayonnaise-type dressings that contribute a large amount of total fat and calories would maintain healthy dietary practices, compared to other foods that do not contain such high amounts of fats and calories in such small serving sizes. Also, there are many foods that are naturally lower in total fat on a weight basis than spreads and mayonnaise-type dressings to which EPA and DHA containing food ingredients could be added; therefore, consumers would have many foods to choose from to obtain the purported health benefit of EPA and DHA. Therefore, FDA has decided to not accept the comment's suggestion, and instead, considers compliance with the "total fat" disqualifying levels as a condition of its enforcement discretion for spreads and mayonnaise-type dressings.

However, FDA does believe that it would be appropriate to consider, as a factor in the exercise of its enforcement discretion, that dietary supplements that weigh equal to or less than 5 g per RACC that exceed the per 50 g total fat disqualifying level (i.e., above 13.0 g of total fat per 50 g), be eligible to bear an omega-3 fatty acid qualified health claim. As explained earlier, most EPA- and DHA-containing dietary supplements are in softgel forms. A serving of fish oil or algal oil dietary supplements in softgels normally contain extremely small amount of total fat (about 0.5 - 2 g of total fat). Liquid forms of fish oils are rare and the serving size is labeled as a teaspoonful. A teaspoonful of fish oil contains about 4.5 g of total fat. FDA is not aware of algal oil dietary supplements in a liquid form. In either softgel or liquid forms, one serving of an EPA- and DHA-containing dietary supplement that weighs equal to or less than 5 g per RACC would provide a very small amount of total fat. It is highly unlikely that individuals would consume 50 g of dietary supplements per day. Therefore, FDA believes that it would be appropriate to consider the exercise of its enforcement discretion for the use of an omega-3 fatty acid qualified health claim for dietary supplements that weigh equal to or less than 5 g per RACC but that exceed the disqualifying level for total fat per 50 g. If the total fat level of dietary supplements that weigh equal to or less than 5 g per RACC exceeds the per 50 g disqualifying level, the disclosure statement (i.e., "See nutrition information for total fat content") required by 21 CFR 101.14(e)(3) must be placed immediately adjacent to and directly beneath the claim, with no intervening material, in the same size, typeface, and contrast as the claim itself. FDA does not intend to exercise its enforcement discretion with respect to all other applicable labeling requirements that apply to dietary supplements, including 21 CFR 101.36(b)(2) that requires dietary supplements to declare the amount of nutrients when the level exceeds the amount that can be declared as zero. Please note that dietary supplements that are not subject to FDA's enforcement discretion that weigh more than 5 g per RACC are subject to the per 50 g total fat disqualifying level, consistent with 21 CFR 101.14(a)(4).

"Saturated Fat" Disqualifying Level

In exercising enforcement discretion for the omega-3 qualified health claim, FDA intends to consider, as a factor in the exercise of its enforcement discretion, the disqualifying saturated fat level, as defined in 21 CFR 101.14(a)(4), for all conventional foods including products that are essentially all fish. FDA believes that almost all products that are essentially all fish do not exceed the saturated fat disqualifying level. FDA also believes that many other conventional foods to which EPA and DHA could be added do not exceed the saturated fat disqualifying level.

The EPA- and DHA-containing dietary supplements generally exceed the saturated fat disqualifying level per 50 g (i.e., above 4.0 g of saturated fat per 50 g). Fish oils contain 10 - 15 g of saturated fat per 50 g (USDA National Nutrient Database for Standard Reference, Release 17). The algal oil used for dietary supplements contains 15 - 20 g of saturated fat per 50 g.[62]

A serving of EPA- and DHA- containing dietary supplements in softgels normally contain about 0.5 - 2 g of total fat. This amount of fish oil or algal oil does not contain more than 1 g of saturated fat. Also, a teaspoon of fish oil contains about 0.9 - 1.4 g of saturated fat, a level that is below the saturated fat disqualifying level per RACC (4 g). Given that the suggested consumption level is so low, it is highly unlikely that individuals would consume 50 g of dietary supplements, which might contain about 10 - 20 g of saturated fat. Because the amount of saturated fat consumed through dietary supplements which weigh equal to or less than 5 g per RACC is small, FDA has decided not to consider, as a factor in the exercise of its enforcement discretion, that such dietary supplements bearing an omega-3 fatty acid qualified health claim meet the per 50 g saturated fat disqualifying level. If the saturated fat level of dietary supplements that weigh equal to or less than 5 g per RACC exceeds the per 50 g disqualifying level, the disclosure statement (i.e., "See nutrition information for saturated fat content") required by §101.14(e)(3) must be placed immediately adjacent to and directly beneath the claim, with no intervening material, in the same size, typeface, and contrast as the claim itself. Dietary supplements that weigh more than 5 g per RACC must comply with the per 50 g saturated fat disqualifying level, consistent with 21 CFR 101.14(a)(4).

"Cholesterol" Disqualifying Level
Products that are Essentially all Fish

As discussed earlier, FDA applies the "extra lean" criterion for cholesterol as a factor in the exercise of its enforcement discretion for the omega-3 fatty acid qualified health claim. The "extra lean" criterion allows more cholesterol per RACC (95 mg per RACC) than does the cholesterol disqualifying level (60 mg per RACC) for products that are essentially all fish. The agency has decided not to consider, as a factor in the exercise of its enforcement discretion, that these products bearing an omega-3 fatty acid qualified health claim meet the cholesterol disqualifying level because, as discussed earlier, observational studies (Albert et al., 1998, 2002; Hu et al., 2002; Mozaffarian et al., 2003) conducted among healthy individuals showed an association of fish intake with reduced risk of CHD. If the cholesterol level of products that are essentially all fish exceed the cholesterol disqualifying level, the disclosure statement (i.e., "See nutrition information for cholesterol content") required by §101.14(e)(3) must be placed immediately adjacent to and directly beneath the claim, with no intervening material, in the same size, typeface, and contrast as the claim itself.

Other Conventional Foods and Dietary Supplements

FDA intends to consider, as a factor in the exercise of its enforcement discretion, the disqualifying cholesterol level, as defined in 21 CFR 101.14(a)(4), for all conventional foods other than products that are essentially all fish and dietary supplements. FDA does not intend to consider, as a factor in the exercise of its enforcement discretion, that dietary supplements weighing equal to or less than 5 g per RACC that bear an omega-3 fatty acid qualified health claim meet the cholesterol disqualifying criteria on a per 50 g basis for the same reasons discussed in the "low cholesterol" criteria in section IV A. If the cholesterol level of dietary supplements that weigh equal to or less than 5 g per RACC exceeds the per 50 g disqualifying level, the disclosure statement (i.e., "See nutrition information for cholesterol content") required by §101.14(e)(3) must be placed immediately adjacent to and directly beneath the claim, with no intervening material, in the same size, typeface, and contrast as the claim itself. Dietary supplements that weigh more than 5 g per RACC must comply with the per 50 g cholesterol disqualifying level, consistent with 21 CFR 101.14(a)(4).

"Sodium" Disqualifying Level

FDA intends to consider, as a factor in the exercise of its enforcement discretion for the use of an omega-3 fatty acid qualified health claim, the sodium disqualifying nutrient level as specified in 21 CFR 101.14(a)(4) for dietary supplements and conventional foods, including products that are essentially all fish.

C. 10 Percent Minimum Nutrient Content Requirement

Under the general requirements for health claims, a conventional food may not bear a health claim unless it contains, prior to any nutrient addition, at least 10 percent of the Daily Value for vitamin A, vitamin C, iron, calcium, protein, or dietary fiber per RACC (see 21 CFR 101.14(e)(6)). The purpose of this provision is to prevent the use of health claims on foods of minimal nutritional value.

Dietary Supplements

The 10 percent minimum nutrient content requirement does not apply to dietary supplements (21 CFR 101.14(e)(6)).

"Products that are Essentially all fish"

The 10% minimum nutrient content requirement per RACC for protein is 5 grams. Products that are essentially all fish contain more than 5 grams of protein per RACC. Thus, FDA believes that such products would qualify for the requirement. FDA intends to consider, as a factor in the exercise of its enforcement discretion, that products that are essentially all fish that bear an omega-3 fatty acid qualified health claim meet the 10 percent minimum nutrient content requirement.

Other Conventional Foods

FDA intends to consider, as a factor in the exercise of its enforcement discretion, that other conventional foods meet the 10 percent minimum nutrient content requirement. A comment requested that FDA eliminate the minimum nutrient content requirement for dressings for salad and mayonnaise-type dressings. These foods are almost completely devoid of the nutrients that are required to be present at 10 percent or more of reference daily intake as specified in 21 CFR 101.14(e)(6). These foods are the type of foods that FDA had in mind when it required the 10 percent minimum nutrient content as a general requirement for health claims because nutritional values are low while fat and calories are high. FDA considers that the presence of an omega-3 qualified health claim on salad dressings and mayonnaise-type dressings that do not meet the 10% minimum nutrient content requirement would be inconsistent with the principle of health claims, i.e., that health claims should be used on foods that help maintain healthy dietary practices. Since there are many conventional foods enriched with EPA and DHA omega-3 fatty acids that could meet the 10 percent minimum nutrient content requirement, FDA believes that there is no need to consider enforcement discretion for a qualified claim on dressings for salad and mayonnaise-type dressings that do not meet the 10 percent minimum nutrient content requirement.

D. Context of a Total Daily Diet

A provision of the general requirements for health claims requires that a health claim enable the public to comprehend the information provided and to understand the relative significance of such information in the context of the total daily diet (see section 403(r)(3)(B)(iii) of the Act (21 U.S.C. 343 (r)(3)(B)(iii) and 21 CFR 101.14(d)(2)(v))). For health claims pertaining to coronary heart disease that are authorized by regulation (e.g., health claims about fruit, vegetables and grain products that contain fiber, particularly soluble fiber, and risk of coronary heart disease (21 CFR 101.77)), FDA requires information relative to a total diet low in saturated fat and cholesterol because this is an essential part of dietary guidance for reducing the risk of CHD.

However, in FDA's previous letter, regarding omega-3 fatty acids and CHD qualified health claims (February 8, 2002 letter[63]), the agency decided that its exercise of enforcement discretion was not contingent on the use of the sentence (i.e., "It is known that diets low in saturated fat and cholesterol may reduce the risk of heart disease.") in connection with the claim. FDA made this decision because the scientific data that the agency relied on did not specifically evaluate whether the potential benefit of consuming EPA and DHA omega-3 fatty acids on CHD risk depends upon subjects consuming diets low in saturated fat and cholesterol. Because FDA is not aware of any new scientific data that might shed light on this subject, the agency has decided to take the same position discussed in the February 8, 2002 letter. Thus, FDA will not consider the exercise of its enforcement discretion to be contingent upon the use of the phrase or sentence relating diets low in saturated fat and cholesterol in the claim.

E. Daily Dietary Intake Needed to Achieve the Claimed Effect

The general requirements for health claims provide that, if the claim is about the effects of consuming the substance at other than decreased dietary levels, the level of the substance must be sufficiently high and in an appropriate form to justify the claim. Where no definition for "high" has been established, the claim must specify the daily dietary intake necessary to achieve the claimed effect (see 21 CFR 101.14(d)(2)(vii)). Several comments stated that 0.5 to 1 g of EPA and DHA are the effective daily dietary intake levels of EPA and DHA in reducing the risk of CHD, and that about one fourth of the amount (100 to 250 mg of EPA and DHA) should be the minimum level of EPA and DHA per RACC necessary to bear the qualified health claim. One comment suggested 32 mg of EPA and DHA as the minimum level of EPA and DHA necessary to bear the qualified health claim.

The minimum daily dietary intake level is based on the total amount of substance consumed in a day (g/day) and is calculated by summing the amount consumed through supplementation with the amount consumed in the diet. However, as concluded in FDA's previous review on omega-3 fatty acids and CHD (October 31, 2000 letter[64]), the agency finds that this provision cannot be applied to the qualified claim for EPA and DHA omega-3 fatty acids and reduced risk of CHD because the scientific evidence for this relationship is not conclusive and does not support the establishment of a recommended daily dietary intake level or even a possible level of effect for the general U.S. population. Therefore, the agency continues to consider any label or labeling suggesting a level of omega-3 fatty acids to be useful in achieving a reduction in the risk of CHD for the general healthy population to be false and misleading under Section 403(a) of the Act.

FDA concludes that the use of EPA and DHA omega-3 fatty acids as dietary supplements and as an ingredient in conventional foods is safe and lawful under 21 CFR 101.14, provided that the daily intakes of EPA and DHA omega-3 fatty acids do not exceed 3 grams per person per day from conventional foods and dietary supplement sources. Further, in order to help ensure that a consumer does not exceed an intake of 3 grams per person per day of EPA and DHA omega-3 fatty acids from consumption of a dietary supplement with the qualified health claim, FDA intends to consider, as a factor in the exercise of its enforcement discretion, that an EPA- and DHA-containing dietary supplement bearing a qualified claim not recommend or suggest in its labeling a daily intake exceeding 2 grams of EPA and DHA.

As previously stated, the agency is encouraging manufacturers to limit the products that bear the qualified health claim for omega-3 fatty acids and reduced risk of CHD to a daily intake of 1 gram. Further, the agency would consider dietary supplements that bear the qualified claim that encourage intakes (in labeling or under ordinary conditions of use) above 2 grams per day to be outside the scope of the agency's consideration of its enforcement discretion. FDA expects EPA and DHA levels of conventional foods enriched with EPA and DHA containing food ingredients not to exceed the maximum use level specified in the menhaden oil GRAS affirmation or the

GRAS notifications (to which FDA did not object) specific to their oil and food category. Also, as explained in the section on safety of foods containing EPA and DHA (see section I.C.), FDA intends to consider, as a factor in the exercise of its enforcement discretion, that conventional foods and dietary supplements that bear an omega-3 fatty acid qualified health claim declare the amount of EPA and DHA per serving in the claim.

V. Fish and Mercury

FDA received a few comments specific to the safety of fish and fish oils. The Martek petition stated that the presence of mercury in fish can harm the developing nervous systems of unborn children, infants, and young children, and therefore, the presence of mercury in fish and fish derivatives needs to be addressed in the health claim. The Martek petition referenced the March 2004 FDA advisory that cautions pregnant women, women who might become pregnant, nursing mothers and young children against the consumption of certain fish, and that suggests limits to weekly intake of other fish and shellfish. Specifically, the Martek petition stated that certain fish (including shark, swordfish, king mackerel, and tile fish) and other fish that similarly become included in a future FDA advisory should be ineligible to bear the proposed health claim. The Martek petition further suggested that when the health claim appears on other fish, it should be accompanied by an advisory statement suggesting a limited weekly intake for a vulnerable population of pregnant women, women of childbearing age, nursing mothers, and young children. In addition, the Martek petition stated that sources of omega-3 fatty acids derived from fish (such as fish oils) should be ineligible for the health claim unless the oil has been tested and found to contain less than 0.025 ppm of mercury. Finally, the Martek petition stated that the presence of mercury may offset the cardio-protective effects of omega-3 fatty acids, and therefore, that the claim would be misleading if it appeared on fish that contained elevated levels of mercury. The Martek petition stated that the mercury specific limitations and the advisory language would be needed to ensure that the claim is truthful and not misleading under sections 403(a) and 201(n) of the Act.

In a comment that you submitted in response to the Martek petition, you concurred with the suggested prohibition of the use of the proposed health claim on shark, king mackerel, swordfish, and tile fish and with the need for an advisory as part of the claim on other fish, but only for those fish that contained 1 ppm total mercury or less. You disagreed with the Martek petition that mercury may diminish the protective effects of omega-3 fatty acids on heart health. Finally, you presented modified language for the proposed advisory statement on other fish and provided a statement for use on omega-3 fatty acid dietary supplements, containing 1 ppm total mercury or less, stating that intake of omega-3 fatty acids from such supplements should be limited to no more than 3000 mg/day. You suggested setting 1 ppm mercury as an eligibility criterion for qualified health claims for all foods and dietary supplements.

Yet another comment asserted that most of the refining techniques ensure the removal of contaminants, such as mercury, from fish oil products, and often achieve levels below the level of detection. The comment asserted that highly refined fish oils are safe to ingest at the recommended levels when consumed as conventional foods or as dietary supplements. FDA is not aware of any contrary information.

However, FDA does question the basis of the Martek petition's assertion that in order to bear omega-3 fatty acid qualified health claims, fish oils have to be tested and confirmed to contain less than 0.025 ppm of mercury, a level the Martek petition claims is the limit of detection for the most sensitive test accepted as standard by the Association of Official Analytical Chemists. Top selling fish oil dietary supplements have been reported not to contain any significant amount of mercury (Foran et al., 2003 and Consumer Reports, 2003) and FDA is not aware of any data that has shown otherwise. Further, FDA notes that in order for conventional foods to bear omega-3 fatty acid qualified health claims, EPA- and DHA-containing food ingredients have to be generally recognized as safe (GRAS). The determination of GRAS includes an evaluation of possible contaminants including mercury. For instance, the menhaden oil GRAS affirmation (21 CFR 185.1472(a)(2)(ix)) sets a limit on mercury content (0.5 ppm) and GRAS notifications for other EPA and DHA containing food ingredients[65] did not raise FDA's concerns for mercury. Given that there are no data showing that the mercury content of fish oils are high and that the Martek petition's reason for setting 0.025 ppm was based upon detection limit rather than effect on health, FDA is not persuaded to adopt the Martek petition's request.

With regard to your comment suggesting setting 1 ppm as an eligibility criterion for conventional foods and dietary supplements, as mentioned previously, FDA does not expect that the mercury content of dietary supplements would be close to 1 ppm. Also, the GRAS notification process for conventional foods ensures that the mercury level specifications for EPA and DHA containing food ingredients are low enough to protect the public health. Therefore, FDA concludes that there is no need for the agency's exercise of enforcement discretion for the omega-3 fatty acid qualified health claim on fish oils to be contingent on additional specifications for mercury.

FDA disagrees with the petitioners' contention that the omega-3 fatty acid qualified health claim should be accompanied by a product label statement about mercury content of fish and possible harmful health effects to the vulnerable population of pregnant women, women who might become pregnant, nursing mothers, and young children. For some time, FDA has been addressing the issue of reducing the exposure to the harmful effects of mercury by communicating with this target population (pregnant women, women who might become pregnant, nursing mothers, and parents of young children) through the use of consumer advisories. The latest consumer advisory was issued in March 2004 jointly by FDA and the Environmental Protection Agency.[66] This advisory includes information about mercury and makes recommendations about the kinds and amount of fish to eat and to avoid.

Agencies are granted broad discretion in determining the means by which to pursue policy goals.[67] Furthermore, the agency believes that the consumer advisory is a preferable method to educate the target population about mercury in fish, for several reasons. First, consumer advisories are communicated to the target population directly.[68] Second, FDA believes that the advisory approach is more effective than a product label statement in relaying the complex messages about mercury in fish and shellfish. For example, the current advisory distinguishes the mercury content in the fish by identifying specifically which fish to eat and not eat and how much fish to eat of the different types. The advisory also identifies which common fish are low in mercury. This level of clarity and detail would be difficult to provide on a product label statement, due to the limited space. Furthermore, confusion could take place when different kinds of label statements are put on different species of commercial fish and not on locally caught fish. Third, a label statement that reaches the public at large can also have unintended adverse public health consequences. FDA focus group results suggest that people who are not in the target audience (i.e., women who are not nursing and not likely to become pregnant, and men) might eat less fish or refrain from eating fish altogether when they receive information about the mercury content of fish and possible harmful health effects to pregnant women, women who might become pregnant, nursing mothers, and young children (ORC Macro, 2003).

Therefore, the statement about possible harmful effects of mercury accompanying the qualified health claim would likely have the effect of negating the qualified health claim. In summary, FDA has decided that it is preferable not to use a label statement about mercury and possible harmful effect to pregnant women, women who might become pregnant, nursing mothers and young children as a condition for the agency's enforcement discretion for the omega-3 fatty acid qualified health claims.

FDA also disagrees with petitioners' suggestion that FDA not allow the use of omega-3 fatty acid qualified health claims on the four fish the FDA advisory warns the target population not to consume. FDA has not issued any advice about the consumption of these fish for the general public, particularly the non-target population (i.e., men, adolescents, women who are not nursing and not likely to become pregnant) and the agency does not believe that it is necessary to prohibit labels of these fish from bearing omega-3 fatty acid qualified health claims.

Finally, FDA disagrees with the assertion in the Martek petition that it would be misleading not to have a statement about mercury's effects on the cardio-protective effects of EPA and DHA omega-3 fatty acids from fish. There are only a few studies on this subject and results are inconsistent. A case-control study by Guallar et al. (2002) showed an association between mercury levels in toenails and increased risk of myocardial infarction. A case-control study within a large prospective cohort, conducted by Yoshizawa et al. (2003) found no association between mercury levels in toenails and CHD risk. After excluding dentists, who were found to have higher levels of mercury in toenails than other study participants, the analysis did not find a significant association between mercury levels in toenails and CHD risk. A cohort study by Salonen et al. (1995) did find an association between mercury levels in hair and increased risk of acute myocardial infarction. But, a case-control study within an ongoing community intervention program on cardiovascular disease and diabetes prevention, conducted by Hallgren et al. (2001), found an association between the concentration of mercury in erythrocytes and decreased risk of CHD. Thus, these observational studies showed inconsistent results regarding the relationship between mercury and CHD. FDA believes that whether mercury has any role in CHD risk is an unanswered scientific question. Consequently, it is not possible to determine whether mercury counteracts the cardio-protective effects of EPA and DHA omega-3 fatty acids from fish. In summary, FDA finds that the Martek assertion that mercury can counteract the beneficial effect of omega-3 fatty acids as speculative, and FDA will not consider, as a factor in the exercise of its enforcement discretion, that foods that bear an omega-3 fatty acid qualified health claim also bear the suggested label statement, "At high levels, mercury may diminish the protective effects of omega-3 fatty acids on heart health."

VI. Conclusions

Based on FDA's consideration of the scientific evidence and other information submitted with your petition, and other pertinent scientific evidence and information, FDA concludes that there is sufficient evidence for a qualified health claim, provided that the qualified claim is appropriately worded so as to not mislead consumers. Thus, FDA will consider exercising enforcement discretion for the following qualified health claim:

> Supportive but not conclusive research shows that consumption of EPA and DHA omega-3 fatty acids may reduce the risk of coronary heart disease. One serving of [Name of the food] provides [ ] gram of EPA and DHA omega-3 fatty acids. [See nutrition information for total fat, saturated fat, and cholesterol content.]

Dietary supplements may declare the amount of EPA and DHA per serving in "Supplement Facts," instead of making the declaration in the claim.

FDA intends to consider exercising enforcement discretion for the above qualified claim when all other factors for enforcement discretion identified in Section IV of this letter are met.

Please note that scientific information is subject to change, as are consumer consumption patterns. FDA intends to evaluate new information that becomes available to determine whether it necessitates a change in this decision. For example, scientific evidence may become available that will support significant scientific agreement or that will no longer support the use of a qualified claim, or that may raise safety concerns about the substance that is the subject of the claim.

Sincerely,

William K. Hubbard
Associate Commissioner for Policy and Planning

REFERENCES

Albert, C.M., C.H. Hennekens, C.J. O'Donnell, U.A. Ajani, V.J. Carey, W.C. Willett., J.N. Ruskin, and J.E. Manson. Fish consumption and risk of sudden cardiac death. *Journal of the American Medical Association.* 1998; 279(1):23-28.

Albert, C.M., H. Campos, M.J. Stampfer, P.M. Ridker, J.E. Manson., W.C. Willett, and J. Ma. Blood levels of long-chain n-3 fatty acids and the risk of sudden death. *The New England Journal of Medicine.* 2002; 346(15):1113-1118.

Angerer, P., W. Kothny, S. Störk, and C. von Schacky. Effect of dietary supplementation with ω-3 fatty acids on progression of atherosclerosis in carotid arteries. *Cardiovascular Research.* 2002; 54(1):183-190.

Bang, H.O., J. Dyerberg, and H.M. Sinclair. The composition of the Eskimo food in north western Greenland. *American Journal of Clinical Nutrition.* 1980;33(12):2657-2661.

Bucher, H.C., P. Hengstler, C. Schindler, and G. Meier. N-3 polyunsaturated fatty acids in coronary heart disease: a meta-analysis of randomized controlled trials. *American Journal of Medicine.* 2002;112(4):298-304.

Burr, M.L., A.M. Fehily, J.F. Gilbert, S. Rogers, R.M. Holliday, P.M. Sweetnam, P.C. Elwood, and N.M. Deadman. Effects of changes in fat, fish, and fibre intakes on death and myocardial reinfarction: Diet and Reinfarction Trial (DART). *Lancet.* 1989;2(8666):757-761.

Burr, M.L., P.M. Sweetham, and A.M. Fehily. Letter to the Editor. Diet and reinfarction. *European Heart Journal.* 1994;15(8):1152-1153.

Connor, W.E. Importance of n-3 fatty acids in health and disease. *American Journal of Clinical Nutrition.* 2000;71(1 Suppl):171S-175S.

Consumer Reports. Omega-3 Oil. Fish or Pills? Pages 30-32, July 2003

de Lorgeril, M., P. Salen, P. Defaye, P. Mabo, and F. Paillard. Dietary prevention of sudden cardiac death. *European Heart Journal.* 2002;23(4):277-285.

Dyerberg, J., H.O. Bang, E. Stoffersen, S. Moncada, and J.R. Vane. Eicosapentaenoic acid and prevention of thrombosis and atherosclerosis? *Lancet.* 1978;2(8081):117-119.

Federal Judicial Center, *Reference Manual on Scientific Evidence*, Second Edition, 2000, page 93

Finnegan, Y.E., A.M. Minihane, E.C. Leigh-Firbank, S. Kew, G.W. Meijer, R. Muggli, P.C. Calder, and C.M. Williams. Plant- and marine-derived n-3 polyunsaturated fatty acids have differential effects on fasting and postprandial blood lipid concentrations and on the susceptibility of LDL to oxidative modification in moderately hyperlipidemic subjects. *American Journal of Clinical Nutrition*. 2003;77(4):783-795.

Foran, S.E., J.G. Flood, and K.B. Lewandrowski. Measurement of mercury levels in concentrated over-the-counter fish oil preparations. Is fish oil healthier than fish? *Arachives of Pathology & Laboratory Medicine*. 2003;127:1603-1605.

Ghafoorunissa, A. Vani, R. Laxmi, and B. Sesikeran. Effects of dietary α-linolenic acid from blended oils on biochemical indices of coronary heart disease in Indians. *Lipids*. 2002;37(11):1077-1086.

Gillum, R.F., M. Mussolino, and J.H. Madans. The relation between fish consumption, death from all causes, and incidence of coronary heart disease. The NHANES I Epidemiologic Follow-up Study. *Journal of Clinical Epidemiology*. 2000;53(3):237-244.

GISSI-Prevenzione Investigators. Dietary supplementation with n-3 polyunsaturated fatty acids and vitamin E after myocardial infarction: results of the GISSI-Prevenzione trial. *Lancet*. 1999; 354:447-455.

Goel, D.P., T.G. Maddaford, and G.N. Pierce. Effects of ω-3 polyunsaturated fatty acids on cardiac sarcolemmal Na+/H+ exchange. *American Journal of Physiology-Heart and Circulatory Physiology*. 2002;283(4):H1688-H1694.

Guallar, E., M.I. Sanz-Gallardo, P. van't Veer, P. Bode, A. Aro, J. Gomez-Aracena, J.D. Kark, R.A. Riemersma, J.M. Martin-Moreno, and F.J. Kok, for the Heavy Metals and Myocardial Infarction Study Group. Mercury, fish oils, and the risk of myocardial infarction. *The New England Journal of Medicine*. 2002;347:1747-1754.

Hallgren, C.G., G. Hallmans, J.H. Jansson, S.L. Marklund, F. Huhtasaari, A. Schütz, U. Strömberg, B. Vessby, and S. Skerfving. Markers of high fish intake are associated with decreased risk of a first myocardial infarction. *British Journal of Nutrition*. 2001;86(3):397-404.

Hu, F.B., L. Bronner, W.C. Willett, M.J. Stampfer, K.M. Rexrode, C.M. Albert, D. Hunter, and J.E. Manson. Fish and ω-3 fatty acid intake and risk of coronary heart disease in women. *Journal of the American Medical Association*. 2002;287(14):1815-1821.

Hu, F.B., E. Cho, K.M. Rexrode, C.M. Albert, and J.E. Manson. Fish and long-chain ω-3 fatty acid intake and risk of coronary heart disease and total mortality in diabetic women. *Circulation*. 2003;107(14):1852-1857.

Institute of Medicine of the National Academies, *Dietary Reference Intakes for Energy, Carbohydrate, Fiber, Fat, Fatty Acids, Cholesterol, Protein and Amino Acids*. Chapter 8, "Dietary Fats: Total Fat and Fatty Acids," and Chapter 11, "Macronutrients and Healthful Diets," (National Academy Press 2002).

Kris-Etherton, P.M., W.S. Harris, and L.J. Appel; American Heart Association. Nutrition Committee. Fish consumption, fish oil, omega-3 fatty acids, and cardiovascular disease. *Circulation.* 2002;106(21):2747-2757.

Krokan, H.E., K.S. Bjerve, and E. Mørk. The enteral bioavailability of eicosapentaenoic acid and docosahexaenoic acid is good from ethyl esters as from glyceryl esters in spite of lower hydrolytic rates by pancreatic lipase in vitro. *Biochimica et Biophysica Acta.* 1993;1168(1):59-67.

Laidlaw, M. and B.J. Holub. Effects of supplementation with fish oil-derived n-3 fatty acids and γ-linolenic acid on circulating plasma lipids and fatty acid profiles in women. *American Journal of Clinical Nutrition.* 2003;77(1):37-42.

Leaf, A., J.X. Kang, Y.F. Xiao, and G.E. Billman. Clinical prevention of sudden cardiac death by n-3 polyunsaturated fatty acids and mechanism of prevention of arrhythmias by n-3 fish oils. *Circulation.* 2003;107(21):2646-2652.

Lemaitre, R.N., I.B. King, D. Mozaffarian, L.H. Kuller, R.P. Tracy, and D.S. Siscovick. n-3 Polyunsaturated fatty acids, fatal ischemic heart disease, and nonfatal myocardial infarction in older adults: the Cardiovascular Health Study. *American Journal of Clinical Nutrition.* 2003; 77(2):319-325.

Leng, G.C., A.J. Lee, F.G. Fowkes, R.G. Jepson, G.D. Lowe, E.R. Skinner, and B.F. Mowat. Randomized controlled trial of gamma-linolenic acid and eicosapentaenoic acid in peripheral arterial disease. *Clinical Nutrition.* 1998;17(6):265-271.

Marchioli, R., F. Barzi, E. Bomba, C. Chieffo, D. Di Gregorio, R. Di Mascio, M.G. Franzosi, E. Geraci, G. Levantesi, A.P. Maggioni, L. Mantini, R.M. Marfisi, G. Mastrogiuseppe, N. Mininni, G.L. Nicolosi, M. Santini, C. Schweiger, L. Tavazzi, G. Tognoni, C. Tucci, and F. Valagussa; GISSI-Prevenzione Investigators. Early protection against sudden death by n-3 polyunsaturated fatty acids after myocardial infarction: time-course analysis of the results of the Gruppo Italiano per lo Studio della Sopravvivenza nell'Infarto Miocardico (GISSI)-Prevenzione. *Circulation.* 2002;105(16):1897-1903.

Maresta, A., M. Balduccelli, E. Varani, M. Marzilli, C. Galli, F. Heiman, M. Lavezzari, E. Stragliotto, and R. De Caterina; ESPRIT Investigators. Prevention of postcoronary angioplasty restenosis by omega-3 fatty acids: main results of the Esapent for Prevention of Restenosis ITalian Study (ESPRIT). *American Heart Journal.* 2002;143(6):E5.

Mozaffarian, D., R.N. Lemaitre, L.H. Kuller, G.L. Burke, R.P. Tracy, and D.S. Siscovick; Cardiovascular Health Study. Cardiac benefits of fish consumption may depend on the type of fish meal consumed: the Cardiovascular Health Study. *Circulation.* 2003;107(10):1372-1377.

Nilsen, D.W., G. Albrektsen, K. Landmark, S. Moen, T. Aarsland, and L. Woie. Effects of a high-dose concentrate of n-3 fatty acids or corn oil introduced early after an acute myocardial infarction on serum triacylglycerol and HDL cholesterol. *American Journal of Clinical Nutrition.* 2001;74(1):50-56.

ORC Macro. *Consumer reactions to the draft advisory on methyl mercury in fish. Focus Group Research.* Summary of key findings. U.S. Food and Drug Administration. March 2003.

Osler, M., A.H. Andreasen, and S. Hoidrup. No inverse association between fish consumption and risk of death from all-causes, and incidence of coronary heart disease in middle-aged, Danish adults. *Journal of Clinical Epidemiology.* 2003;56(3):274-279.

Pepe, S. and P.L. McLennan. Cardiac membrane fatty acid composition modulates myocardial oxygen consumption and postischemic recovery of contractile function. *Circulation.* 2002; 105(19):2303-2308.

Rissanen, T., S. Voutilainen, K. Nyyssönen, T.A. Lakka, and J.T. Salonen. Fish oil-derived fatty acids, docosahexaenoic acid and docosapentaenoic acid, and the risk of acute coronary events: the Kuopio Ischaemic Heart Disease Risk Factor Study. *Circulation.* 2000;102(22):2677-2679.

Salonen, J.T., K. Seppänen, K. Nyyssönen, H. Korpela, J. Kauhanen, M. Kantola, J. Tuomilehto, H. Esterbauer, F. Tatzber, and R. Salonen. Intake of mercury from fish, lipid peroxidation, and the risk of myocardial infarction and coronary, cardiovascular, and any death in Eastern Finnish men. *Circulation.* 1995;91:645-655.

Sacks, F.M., P.H. Stone, C.M. Gibson, D.I. Silverman, B. Rosner, and R.C. Pasternak. Controlled trial of fish oil for regression of human coronary atherosclerosis. HARP Research Group. *Journal of the American College of Cardiology.* 1995;25(7):1492-1498.

Singh, R.B., M.A. Niaz, J.P. Sharma, R. Kumar, V. Rastogi, and M. Moshiri. Randomized, double-blind, placebo-controlled trial of fish oil and mustard oil in patients with suspected acute myocardial infarction: the Indian Experiment of Infarct Survival-4. *Cardiovascular Drugs and Therapy.* 1997;11(3):485-491.

Siscovick, D.S., R.N. Lemaitre, and D. Mozaffarian. The fish story: a diet-heart hypothesis with clinical implications: n-3 polyunsaturated fatty acids, myocardial vulnerability, and sudden death. *Circulation.* 2003;107(21):2632-2634.

Spilker, B. *Guide to Clinical Studies.* Raven Press, New York, New York, 1991.

Thies, F., J.M. Garry, P. Yaqoob, K. Rerkasem, J. Williams, C.P. Shearman, P.J. Gallagher, P.C. Calder, and R.F. Grimble. Association of n-3 polyunsaturated fatty acids with stability of atherosclerotic plaques: a randomized controlled trial. *Lancet.* 2003;361(9356):477-485.

Torres, I.C., L. Mira, C.P. Ornelas, and A. Melim. Study of the effects of dietary fish intake on serum lipids and lipoproteins in two populations with different dietary habits. *British Journal of Nutrition.* 2000;83(4):371-379.

United States Department of Agriculture and United States Department of Health and Human Services. *Nutrition and Your Health: Dietary Guidelines for Americans.* Fifth Edition, 2000. Home and Garden Bulletin No. 232, 2000.

United States Department of Health and Human Services. *Detection, Evaluation, and Treatment of High Blood Cholesterol in Adults* (Adult Treatment Panel III). Executive Summary. NIH Publication No. 01-3670. 2001.

von Schacky, C., P. Angerer, W. Kothny, K. Theisen, and H. Mudra. The effect of dietary ω-3 fatty acids on coronary atherosclerosis. A randomized, double-blind, placebo-controlled trial. *Annals of Internal Medicine.* 1999;130(7):554-562.

Woodman, R.J., T.A. Mori, V. Burke, I.B. Puddey, G.F. Watts, and L.J. Beilin. Effects of purified eicosapentaenoic and docosahexaenoic acids on glycemic control, blood pressure, and serum lipids in type 2 diabetic patients with treated hypertension. *American Journal of Clinical Nutrition.* 2002;76(5):1007-1015.

Yoshizawa, K., E.B. Rimm, J.S. Morris, V.L. Spate, C.C. Hsieh, D. Spiegelman, M.J. Stampfer, and W.C.Willett. Mercury and the risk of coronary heart disease in men. *The New England Journal of Medicine.* 2002;347:1755-1760.

ENDNOTES

[1]   A letter from Christine J. Lewis, Ph.D., FDA to Jonathan W. Emord, Esq., Emord & Associates, P.C., "Letter Regarding Dietary Supplement Health Claim for Omega-3 Fatty Acids and Coronary Heart Disease" (Docket No. 91N-0103), October 31, 2000. http://www.cfsan.fda.gov/~dms/ds-ltr11.html.

[2]   A letter from Christine J. Lewis, Ph.D., FDA to Jonathan W. Emord, Esq., Emord & Associates, P.C., "Letter Clarifying Conditions for a Dietary Supplement Health Claim for Omega-3 Fatty Acids and Coronary Heart Disease" (Docket No. 91N-0103), February 16, 2001. http://www.cfsan.fda.gov/~dms/ds-ltr20.html.

[3]   A letter from Christine J. Taylor, Ph.D., FDA to Jonathan W. Emord, Esq., Emord & Associates, P.C., "Letter Responding to a Request to Reconsider the Qualified Claim for Dietary Supplement Health Claim for Omega-3 Fatty Acids and Coronary Heart Disease" (Docket No. 91N-0103), February 8, 2002. http://www.cfsan.fda.gov/~dms/ds-ltr28.html.

[4]   "Interim Procedures for Qualified Health Claims in the Labeling of Conventional Human Food and Human Dietary Supplements" that published on July 10, 2003. http://www.cfsan.fda.gov/~dms/nuttf-e.html.

[5]   See footnote 1.

[6]   See footnote 2.

[7]   See footnote 3.

[8]   This guidance published on July 10, 2003. http://www.cfsan.fda.gov/~dms/nuttf-b.html.

[9]   A meta-analysis is the process of systematically combining and evaluating the results of clinical trials that have been completed or terminated (i.e., primary reports) (Spilker, 1991). FDA uses meta-analyses to identify relevant primary reports, which the Agency then evaluates individually.

[10]   Review articles summarize the findings of primary reports. FDA uses review articles to identify primary reports that are relevant for review. FDA also uses review articles to identify information that is useful to understand the scientific issues about the substance-disease relationship (i.e., used as background information).

[11]   The physiology of animals is different than that of humans, thus animals often respond differently to dietary interventions compared to humans.

[12]   In vitro studies are conducted in an artificial environment and cannot account for a multitude of normal physiological processes such as digestion, absorption, distribution, and metabolism that affect how humans respond to the consumption of foods and dietary substances. Therefore, in vitro studies generally are not able to provide scientific evidence about the relationship between a substance and disease risk.

[13]   Angerer et al., 2002; Burr et al., 1989; GISSI et al., 1999; Marchioli et al., 2002; Maresta, et al., 2002; Singh et al., 1997.

[14]   Albert et al., 1998; Albert et al., 2002; Hallgren et al., 2001; Hu et al., 2002; Hu et al., 2003; Lamaitre et al., 2003; Mozaffarian et al., 2003; Rissanen et al., 2000.

[15]   Connor, 2000; de Lorgeril et al., 2002; Leaf et al., 2003.

[16]   Kris-Etherton et al., 2002.

[17]   Siscovick et al., 2003.

[18]   Bucher et al., 2002.

[19]   Bang et al., 1980.

[20]   Dyerberg et al., 1978; Goel et al., 2002; Pepe and McLennan, 2002.

[21]   Finnegan et al., 2003; Ghafoorunissa et al., 2002; Laidlaw and Holub 2003; Thies et al., 2003; Woodman et al., 2002.

[22]   Leng et al., 1998.

[23]   Nilsen et al. 2001.

[24]   Gillum et al., 2000; Osler et al., 2003; Torres et al., 2000.

[25]   Institute of Medicine, 2002.

[26]   U.S. Department of Agriculture, Agricultural Research Service. 2004. USDA National Nutrient Database for Standard Reference, Release 17 (http://www.nal.usda.gov/fnic/foodcomp/Data/SR17/sr17.html).

[27]   Summary of all GRAS notices. http://www.cfsan.fda.gov/ ~rdb/opa-gras.html.

[28]   Institute of Medicine of the National Academies. Dietary Reference Intakes. Energy, Carbohydrate, Fiber, Fat, Fatty Acids, Cholesterol, Protein, and Amino Acids. Part 2. Pages E-13, E-14. http://www.nap.edu/books/0309085373/html/.

[29]   Conventional foods enriched with EPA and DHA containing food ingredients are not included in the estimates.

[30]   See footnote 1.

[31]   National Heart, Blood and Lung Institute (NHLBI), Heart and Blood Vessel Diseases (http://www.nhlbi.nih.gov/health/ dci/Diseases/Atherosclerosis/Atherosclerosis_WhatIs.html) and National Cholesterol Education Program, Page 3 (U.S. Department of

Health and Human Services, 2001, http://www.nhlbi.nih.gov/ guidelines/cholesterol/atp_iii.htm).

[32]   See footnote 1.

[33]   Albert et al., 1998; Burr et al., 1994 (also Burr et al., 1989); GISSI-Prevenzione Investigators,1999; Singh et al., 1997.

[34]   Angerer et al., 2002; Marchioli et al., 2002; Maresta et al., 2002.

[35]   Finnegan et al., 2003; Ghafoorunissa et al., 2002; Laidlaw and Holub 2003; Thies et al., 2003; Woodman et al., 2002.

[36]   Leng et al., 1998.

[37]   Nilsen et al. 2001.

[38]   Neither the patient/subject nor the investigator is aware of which treatment the patient/subject is receiving (Spilker, 1991).

[39]   FDA considers the subjects in this study to be representative of the general population because they did not have CHD and the physiological responses to omega-3 fatty acids is the same in hyperlipidemics and normolipidemics (reviewed in the 2000 letter). .

[40]   FDA considered this study relevant to its review because the bioavailability and distribution of EPA ethyl ester and DHA ethyl esters are equivalent to the natural forms of EPA and DHA from fish oil (Krokan, et al., 1993).

[41]   Diabetes is a risk factor for CHD (What Makes a Heart Attach More Likely? National Institutes of Health, National Heart, Lung, and Blood   Institute (http://www.nhlbi.nih.gov/health/dci/Diseases/HeartAttack/heartattac k_risk.html). FDA considers this study on diabetics relevant to its review for establishing the substance-disease relationship because: (1) the diabetic study population did not have CHD and; (2) omega-3 fatty acids affect blood pressure in diabetics and healthy individuals similarly (Evidence Report/Technology Assessment: Number 94, Effects of Omega-3 Fatty Acids on Cardiovascular Disease, Agency for Healthcare Research and Quality, March 2004, page 63-64, http://www.ahrq.gov/clinic/ evrptfiles.htm#o3cardio).

[42]   Hu et al., 2002; Hu et al., 2003; Mozaffarian et al., 2003; Rissanen et al., 2000.

[43]   Gillum et al., 2000; Osler et al., 2003.

[44]   Albert et al., 2002; Hallgren et al., 2001; Lamaitre et al., 2003.

[45]   Torres et al., 2000.

[46]   Gillum et al., 2000; Osler et al., 2003.

[47] Not all fish contain significant amounts of EPA and DHA omega-3 fatty acids (see footnote 26).

[48] Albert et al., 1998, 2002 ; Hallgren et al., 2001; Hu et al., 2002 ; Hu et al., 2003; Lamaitre et al.,2003; Mozaffarian et al., 2003 ; Rissanen et al., 2000; Torres et al., 2000.

[49] Quintiles are values that divide a sample of data into five groups containing (as far as possible) equal numbers of observations.

[50] DPA, docosapentaenoic acid, is formed from EPA and is converted to DHA.

[51] Ischemic heart disease is a form of coronary heart disease (CHD).

[52] A method of dietary assessment in which subjects are asked to recall how frequently certain foods were consumed during a specified period of time.

[53] Dietary Reference Intakes for Energy, Carbohydrate, Fiber, Fat, Fatty Acids, Cholesterol, Protein, and Amino Acids, Part 2, Chapter 11, Page 11-40 (Institutes of the Medicine of the National Academies, 2002).

[54] Guidance for Industry: Significant Scientific Agreement in the Review of Health Claims for Conventional Foods and Dietary Supplements, December 22, 1999 (http://www.cfsan.fda.gov/ ~dms/ssaguide.html). .

[55] See footnote 1.

[56] Telephone communication with Martin J. Hahn on August 24, 2004.

[57] See footnote 1.

[58] See footnote 2.

[59] See footnote 3.

[60] See footnote 56.

[61] See footnote 56.

[62] See footnote 56.

[63] See footnote 3.

[64] See footnote 1.

[65] See footnote 27.

[66] U.S. Department of Health and Human Services and U.S. Environmental Protection Agency, "What You Need to Know About Mercury in Fish and Shellfish, 2004 EPA and FDA Advice For: Women Who Might Become Pregnant, Women Who are Pregnant, Nursing Mothers, Young Children." March 2004. http://www.cfsan.fda.gov/~dms/admehg3.html.

[67] See, e.g., UAW v. Chao, 361 F.3d 249 (3rd Cir. 2004), (court deferred to OSHA's decision to pursue various non-regulatory measures, such

as non-mandatory guidelines and educational programs, rather than to promulgate a rule limiting worker exposure to metalworking fluids, which were acknowledged by the court to have debilitating health effects); CFA v. CPSC, 990 F.2d 1298 (DC Cir. 1993), (court deferred to CPSC's decision to negotiate a comprehensive consent decree with vehicle manufacturers and dealer monitoring agreements, rather than to promulgate a rule banning the sale of all-terrain vehicles for use by children under the age of sixteen. The court stated: "We accord due respect, moreover, to an agency's selection of means for pursuing policy goals. Such choices implicate the allocation of scarce administrative resources; they involve forecasts about the consequences of proposed regulatory actions and other matters the agency ordinarily is best equipped to judge.").

[68]   For instance, with regard to the mercury in fish advisory, the agency is targeting mailings about the advisory to appropriate health professionals, e.g., obstetrician - gynecologists. The agency is also targeting the appropriate media, e.g., women's magazines, as well as professional health organizations that deal with pregnant women, women who might become pregnant, nursing mothers and young children.

LETTER RESPONDING TO HEALTH CLAIM PETITION DATED NOVEMBER 3, 2003 (MARTEK PETITION): OMEGA-3 FATTY ACIDS AND REDUCED RISK OF CORONARY HEART DISEASE (DOCKET NO. 2003Q-0401)

Mr. Martin J. Hahn
Hogan & Hartson, L.L.P.
Columbia Square
555 Thirteenth Street, NW
Washington, DC 20004-1109

RE: Health Claim Petition: Omega-3 Fatty Acids and Reduced Risk of Coronary Heart Disease (Docket No. 2003Q-0401)

Dear Mr. Hahn:

This letter responds to the qualified health claim petition dated November 3, 2003, submitted to the Food and Drug Administration (FDA or the agency), on behalf of Martek Biosciences Corporation (Martek petition) in accordance with the interim procedures for review of qualified health claims described in FDA's July 10, 2003 guidance for procedures on qualified health claims.[1] You submitted the petition as a comment to a petition from Jonathan W. Emord. Mr. Emord submitted the petition on behalf of Wellness Lifestyles, Inc. and Life Extension Foundation Buyers Club (collectively, the Wellness petition).

Your petition requested an extension of the existing omega-3 fatty acids and coronary heart disease (CHD) dietary supplement qualified health claim (a letter dated October 31, 2000,[2] a letter dated February 16, 2001,[3] a letter dated February 8, 2002[4]) to conventional foods including foods fortified with omega-3 fatty acids (specifically eicosapentaenoic acid (EPA) and docosahexaenoic acid (DHA)). Your petition proposed the model health claim: "A growing body of scientific literature suggests that higher intakes of the omega-3 fatty acids DHA and EPA may afford some degree of protection against coronary heart disease." For fish and shellfish, the petition proposed additional statements about potential risks of methylmercury. In your supplemental submission dated April 5, 2004, you requested modification of these statements.

FDA received the Wellness petition on June 23, 2003, for review under the standard health claim petition review process described in Section 403(r)(4) and 403 (r)(5)(D) of the Federal Food Drug and Cosmetic Act (the Act) (21 U.S.C. §§ 343(r)(4) and 343(r)(5)(D)). The Wellness petition requested that the agency authorize a health claim characterizing the relationship between omega-3 fatty acids (specifically EPA and DHA) and reduced risk of CHD. The Wellness petition requested that the disclaimer[4] on the existing omega-3 fatty acids and CHD dietary supplement health claim be removed and that claim be extended to omega-3 containing foods. After corresponding with FDA, the petitioners elected to have their petition processed as a qualified health claim petition. FDA filed the Wellness petition on September 3, 2003 as a qualified health claim petition and posted the petition on the FDA website for a 60 day comment period, consistent with the interim procedures.

Because the substance and disease and the request for an extension of the existing omega-3 and CHD qualified health claim were the same in your petition and the Wellness petition, FDA consolidated the petitions in the same docket (Docket No. 2003Q-0401).

The agency received several comments on the petitions. You submitted two comments, one of which was a petition. Other comments were from industry, a professional organization, and an individual. The comments addressed various issues including the substance of the claim, mercury content in fish, safe upper limit of EPA and DHA, minimum effective levels of EPA and DHA, disqualifying nutrient levels, minimum nutrient content requirement, and claim statements. All support extending the omega-3 fatty acids and CHD qualified health claim to conventional foods. FDA considered the relevant comments in its evaluation of this petition.

This letter sets forth the basis of FDA's determination that the current evidence for the proposed health claim is appropriate for consideration for a qualified health claim on conventional foods and dietary supplements. This letter also sets out the factors that FDA intends to consider for the exercise of its enforcement discretion for a qualified health claim, for both conventional foods and dietary supplements, with respect to consumption of EPA and DHA omega-3 fatty acids and a reduced risk of coronary heart disease. This letter is an update to the previous letters on the use of a qualified health claim on EPA and DHA omega-3 fatty acid dietary supplements and coronary heart disease risk (the October 31, 2000 letter,[5] the February 16, 2001 letter,[6] and the February 8, 2002 letter[7]) and provides FDA's current thinking with respect to the use of this qualified health claim on both dietary supplements and conventional foods. Throughout the text of this letter, the phrase "omega-3 fatty acid qualified health claim" will be used to refer to the qualified health claim about the consumption of EPA and DHA omega-3 fatty acids and a reduced risk of coronary heart disease.

I. Overview of Data and Eligibility for a Qualified Health Claim

In a review of a qualified health claim, FDA considers the data and information provided in the petition, in addition to other data and information available to the agency that may assist in its review of the relationship between the substance and the disease or health-related condition. Consistent with its guidance entitled "Interim Evidence-based Ranking System for Scientific Data,"[8] the agency evaluates the scientific studies to determine what studies are pertinent to its review in evaluating the relationship. The agency may conclude that certain design flaws in a study are so significant that the study may not be helpful to the agency's decision about whether the particular study supports a relationship. Such design flaws may include the lack of a control group or the lack of any analysis of the data (Spilker et al., 1991; Federal Judicial Center, 2000).

In addition to human studies, FDA also considers other data and information in its review, such as meta-analyses,[9] review articles,[10] and animal[11] and *in vitro*[12] studies. These other types of data and information are useful in assisting the agency with an understanding of the scientific issues about a disease or health-related condition, but generally do not themselves establish a health claim relationship in the absence of supporting human intervention or observational data.

After the agency decides what scientific studies are relevant to its review about whether there is evidence to support a relationship between a substance and a disease or health-related condition, (i.e., what studies to rate based on study quality), the agency categorizes these studies into: (1) the most persuasive studies, which are studies designed to evaluate whether there is a relationship between the substance and disease outcome (e.g., intervention studies that manipulate the intake level of the substance while controlling for other factors that can affect disease risk reduction and/or; (2) less persuasive studies (e.g., studies that my have design flaws that make them less reliable in evaluating a substance/disease relationship or less applicable to the U.S. population (conducted in countries where usual intakes of the substance is much lower or higher than in the U.S.). The most persuasive studies are given the greatest consideration. FDA rates the most and less persuasive studies for quality. Scientific quality is based on several criteria including study population, intervention design (e.g., presence of a placebo control), data collection (e.g., dietary assessment method), statistical analysis, and outcome measures. For example, if the scientific study adequately addressed all or most of the above criteria, it would receive a high quality rating. Lower quality ratings (e.g., moderate and low) would be given based on the extent of the deficiencies or uncertainties in the quality criteria.

Collectively, FDA then rates the strength of the total body of evidence that it determines is relevant to its review, using criteria such as the study type (e.g., intervention), quality, quantity (number of the various types of studies and sample sizes), and consistency of the results. Based on the totality of the scientific evidence, FDA determines whether such evidence is credible to support the substance/disease relationship, and if so, then determines the ranking that reflects the level of comfort among qualified scientists that such a relationship is scientifically valid.

The Martek petition cited 42 publications as evidence to substantiate the relationship for this claim. These publications consisted 6 intervention studies on EPA and DHA omega-3 fatty acids and CHD,[13] 7 observational studies on EPA and DHA omega-3 fatty acids and CHD,[14] 5 studies on alpha linoleic acid (ALA) and CHD,[15] 13 review articles,[16] 2 meta-analyses,[17] 1 position paper,[18] 4 editorial comments,[19] 2 chapters from the IOM Report,[20] 2 studies on the safety of fish and fish oils,[21] and 1 abstract.[22]

The agency did not consider all the publications cited in the Martek petition to be pertinent to its review of this substance/disease relationship. While useful for background information, the review articles, position paper, editorial comments, meta-analyses and abstract did not contain sufficient information on the individual studies reviewed and therefore FDA could not determine their pertinence regarding factors such as the study population characteristics or the composition of the products used (e.g., food, dietary supplement); similarly, the lack of detailed information on the studies summarized in the review articles, position paper, editorial comments, meta-analyses and abstract did not allow FDA to determine if the studies are flawed in critical elements such as its design, execution, and data analysis. FDA must review the scientific quality of a study to determine whether credible conclusions can be drawn from it.

In addition to the studies in your petition that the agency considered, FDA considered an additional 7 intervention studies (5 from the Wellness petition[23]; 1 from a comment [24]; 1 identified by FDA through a literature search[25]), and 4 observational studies from the Wellness petition.[26]

A. Substance

A health claim characterizes the relationship between a substance and a disease or health-related condition (21 CFR 101.14(a)(1)). A substance means a specific food or component of food (21 CFR 101.14(a)(2)). The petitions identified the omega-3 fatty acids, eicosapentaenoic acid (EPA) and docosahexaenoic acid (DHA), as the substance for the proposed claim. EPA and DHA are components of some fatty fish (primarily cold water fish),[27] fish oils, other foods (e.g., seaweed), dietary supplements, and food ingredients (e.g., algal oils). Therefore, the agency concludes that the substances, EPA and DHA omega-3 fatty acids, identified in the petition are components of food and therefore meet the definition of substance in the health claim regulation (21 CFR 101.14(a)(2)).

B. Disease or Health-Related Condition

A disease or health-related condition means damage to an organ, part, structure, or system of the body such that it does not function properly, or a state of health leading to such dysfunctioning (21 CFR 101.14(a)(5)). The petition has identified coronary heart disease (CHD) as the disease for the proposed claim. The agency concludes that CHD is a disease and therefore that the petitioner has satisfied the requirement in 21 CFR 101.14(a)(5).

C. Safety Review

Under 21 CFR 101.14(b)(3)(ii), if the substance is to be consumed at other than decreased dietary levels, the substance must be a food or a food ingredient or a component of a food ingredient whose use at levels necessary to justify a claim must be demonstrated by the proponent of the claim, to FDA's satisfaction, to be safe and lawful under applicable food safety provisions of the Federal Food, Drug, and Cosmetic Act.

The Wellness petition stated that omega-3 fatty acids, as EPA and DHA, have been a naturally occurring ingredient in foods consumed safely in the United States prior to January 1, 1958, and that there is no evidence that when consumed either in foods or as dietary supplements there is a cumulative effect in the diet that is unsafe. The Martek petition stated that omega-3 fatty acids occur in conventional foods with a long history of safe use, such as fish, and are generally recognized as safe (GRAS) when used as direct food ingredients intended to increase omega-3 fatty acids. Some comments to the petition expressed an interest in using the omega-3 fatty acid qualified health claim for foods that contain EPA and DHA as a food ingredient from sources including fish oil and algal oil.

In order to meet the safe and lawful requirement for health claims (21 CFR 101.14(b)(3)(ii)), the use of EPA and DHA omega-3 fatty acid, when used in conventional food or as a dietary supplement at levels necessary to justify the claim, must be demonstrated, to FDA's satisfaction, to be safe and lawful. FDA evaluates whether the substance is "safe and lawful" under the applicable food safety provisions of the Act. For conventional foods, this evaluation involves considering whether the ingredient that is the source of the substance is GRAS, approved as a food additive, or authorized by a prior sanction issued by FDA (see 21 CFR 101.70(f)). Dietary ingredients in dietary supplements, however, are not subject to the food additive provisions of the act (see section 201(s)(6) of the Act (21 U.S.C. § 321(s)(6)). Rather, they are subject to the adulteration provisions in section 402 of the Act (21 U.S.C. 342) and, if applicable, the new dietary ingredient provisions in section 413 of the Act (21 U.S.C. 350b), which pertain to dietary ingredients that were not marketed in the United States before October 15, 1994. The term "dietary ingredient" is defined in section 201(ff)(1) of the act and includes vitamins; minerals; herbs and other botanicals; dietary substances for use by man to supplement the diet by increasing the total daily intake; and concentrates, metabolites, constituents, extracts, and combinations of the preceding types of ingredients.

In 1997, FDA affirmed, as GRAS, menhaden oil as a direct human food ingredient with specific limitations of use to ensure that the total daily intake of EPA and DHA would not exceed 3.0 grams per person per day (g/p/d) (62 FR 30751; June 5, 1997; 21 CFR184.1472). EPA and DHA are the major omega-3 fatty acids in fish oil and together comprise about 20 percent by weight of menhaden oil. FDA established maximum use levels of menhaden oil in certain foods because of concerns over possible adverse effects of fish oil consumption on bleeding time, glycemic control, and LDL cholesterol (62 FR 30751 at 30757; June 5, 1997). In 2002, FDA published a proposed rule to reallocate the uses of menhaden oil in conventional food, while maintaining the total daily intake of EPA and DHA from menhaden oil at a level not exceeding 3.0 g/p/d (67 FR 8744; February 26, 2002). FDA placed specific limitations, including the category of foods, the functional use of the ingredient, and the level of use, to ensure that the consumption of EPA and DHA from conventional food sources would not exceed 3.0 g/p/d. FDA then published a tentative final rule (69 FR 2313; January 15, 2004) to additionally require that menhaden oil not be used as an ingredient in foods in combination with other added oil that is a significant source of EPA and DHA to ensure that total intake from conventional food sources do not exceed 3.0 g/p/d.

In addition, FDA has not objected to certain GRAS notifications for additional sources of EPA and DHA as food ingredients (fish oils other than menhaden oil) (GRAS Notice Nos: GRN000097, GRN000102, GRN000105, GRN000109, GRN 000137, GRN000138).[28] These GRAS notices proposed maximum use levels consistent with those specified in the tentative final rule affirming, as GRAS, menhaden oil as a direct human food ingredient with specific limitations of use.

FDA has also responded without objection to a GRAS notification on algal oil DHA from Martek Biosciences Corporation. Martek estimated that the use of algal oil in a number of food categories at the maximum proposed use levels would result in a mean exposure of no more than 1.5 grams of DHA per day (GRAS Notice No. GRN000137).

The mean exposure to EPA and DHA from menhaden oil in all conventional food categories is estimated to be 2.7 g/p/d (67 FR 8744 at

8746; February 26, 2002). This is a conservative estimate with substantial margin for safety, and the agency believes, consistent with its prior decision on the use of a qualified health claim for DHA and EPA omega-3 fatty acids (October 31, 2000 letter), that the addition of menhaden oil to food products has not come close to this conservative mean estimate exposure. FDA further believes that the GRAS uses for which it received a GRAS notification for other sources of EPA and DHA omega-3 fatty acids also provide conservative estimates of exposure and that the addition of these EPA and DHA sources to food products do not come close to the conservative mean estimates. Not all foods in the marketplace within those permitted food categories would contain menhaden oil or other sources of EPA and DHA omega-3 fatty acids that substitute for other edible fat or oil. Also, because not all foods that a consumer eats every day would contain menhaden or other EPA and DHA oil used as a substitute oil, the actual total daily intakes of EPA and DHA from menhaden or other EPA and DHA oil for an average person should be significantly below 3.0 g/p/d (67 FR 8744 at 8746; February 26, 2002).

It is difficult to estimate the actual total consumption of EPA and DHA. The Continuing Survey of Food Intakes by Individuals (1994-1996, 1998)[29] estimated EPA and DHA intakes from conventional foods.[30] The 50th percentile intake of EPA and DHA from the survey was between 0.06 g and 0.07 g for adult women and 0.07 g and 0.1 g for adult men. The 90th percentile intake was between 0.18 g and 0.22 g for women and between 0.20 g and 0.43 g for men. Thus, EPA and DHA consumption from conventional foods in the United States is low. FDA is not aware of any nationally representative consumption data on EPA and DHA from dietary supplements. In the October 31, 2000 letter, FDA expressed concern about the exposure to EPA and DHA omega-3 fatty acids potentially exceeding 3.0 g/p/d if a qualified health claim were to appear on dietary supplements. This concern was due to conventional foods containing omega-3 fatty acids that were on the market; the use of structure/function claims on products containing EPA and DHA omega-3 fatty acids, which may promote product purchase; and dietary supplements that FDA found in the marketplace that contained significant amounts of EPA and DHA.

With this letter, the requested use of this qualified health claim is now extended to conventional foods. The agency believes that there is likely to be some increased consumption of EPA and

DHA omega-3 fatty acids based on conventional foods that bear the qualified health claim; however, the amounts of EPA and DHA that can be used and the foods in which such food ingredients can be safely used are limited. The agency has established specific limitations of use under its menhaden oil GRAS rule (62 FR 30751; June 5, 1997), proposed and tentatively finalized reallocation of the use of menhaden oil without changing total exposure levels (67 FR 8744; February 26, 2002, 69 FR 2313; January 15, 2004). Also, manufacturers that have submitted GRAS notifications for other sources, to which the agency has not objected, have established conditions of use similar to those in the menhaden oil GRAS rule.

In the October 31, 2000 letter,[31] FDA stated that a consumer could consume nearly 1 gram of EPA and DHA per day in the diet from conventional foods. The agency is uncertain about how much consumers will increase their intake of EPA and DHA omega-3 fatty acids from EPA and DHA containing conventional foods and dietary supplements due to the extended use of the qualified health claim. In order to help consumers gauge their total intake of EPA and DHA and to provide them a way to keep their intake of EPA and DHA within 3 grams per day, FDA intends to consider, as a factor in the exercise of its enforcement discretion, that conventional foods and dietary supplements that bear an omega-3 fatty acid qualified health claim declare the amount of EPA and DHA per serving in the claim. FDA recommends that the information on EPA and DHA content for use in a qualified health claim for EPA and DHA omega-3 fatty acids and reduced risk of CHD be presented in a manner that is consistent with FDA's guidance entitled, "FDA Nutrition Labeling Manual--A Guide for Developing and Using Data Bases." You may contact CFSAN's Office of Nutritional Products, Labeling, and Dietary Supplements (ONPLDS) for further information. The dietary supplement may declare the amount of EPA and DHA per serving in "Supplement Facts," instead of making the declaration in the claim. Also, to ensure further that consumers do not exceed a 3.0 g/p/d intake, FDA will educate consumers not to exceed 3.0 g/p/d from all food and dietary supplement sources through print and web outreach information. Further, FDA intends to consider, as a factor in the exercise of its enforcement discretion, that dietary supplements not recommend or suggest in labeling that consumers ingest more than 2 grams of EPA and DHA per day. FDA encourages manufacturers to limit their dietary supplement products bearing the qualified health claim to products recommending or suggesting daily intake of 1 gram or less of EPA and DHA omega-3 fatty acids.

Based on the data and information that FDA considered, which includes data and information that FDA relied upon in reaching its conclusions about the safety of EPA and DHA omega-3 fatty acids in its GRAS affirmation of menhaden oil, the data and information in the 1991 proposed (56 FR 60663; November 27, 1991) and 1993 final rules (58 FR 2683; January 6, 1993), and its current scientific literature review for other possible safety concerns, FDA concludes that the use of EPA and DHA omega-3 fatty acids used as a GRAS ingredient, consistent with FDA's GRAS rule for menhaden oil and GRAS notifications to which FDA did not object, and the use as a dietary supplement is safe and lawful under 21 CFR 101.14 provided that daily intakes of EPA and DHA omega-3 fatty acids from conventional food and dietary supplement sources do not exceed 3.0 g/p/d. In section IV, FDA sets forth factors under which it plans to exercise enforcement discretion for EPA and DHA containing conventional foods and dietary supplements bearing the qualified claim, to ensure, among other things, that such use will be safe.

II. The Agency's Consideration of a Qualified Health Claim

FDA has identified the following endpoints to use in identifying CHD risk reduction for purposes of a health claim evaluation for EPA and DHA omega-3 fatty acids: Coronary events (MI, ischemia), cardiovascular death, atherosclerosis, and high blood pressure. Artherosclerosis is the underlying cause of CHD, which can lead to the signs of CHD including coronary events (MI, ischemia) and cardiovascular death.[32] High blood pressure, serum total cholesterol, serum LDL-cholesterol, and serum HDL-cholesterol are considered as surrogate endpoints for CHD.[33] However, FDA concluded in its October 31, 2000 letter[34] that omega-3 fatty acids do not affect serum cholesterol levels (total, LDL, HDL). To evaluate the potential effects of EPA and DHA omega-3 fatty acid consumption on CHD risk, FDA considered coronary events (myocardial infarction (MI), ischemia), cardiovascular death, atherosclerosis, and high blood pressure as indicators or predictors of disease.

In considering the qualified health claim for EPA and DHA omega-3 fatty acid dietary supplements in October 2000, FDA focused on human data that had become available since FDA's 1991-93 review and on human studies that quantitatively measured or estimated the omega-3 fatty acid intakes in relation to a direct measure of CHD risk or a surrogate endpoint for CHD risk. Several, but not all, of the studies[35] that FDA had considered in its October 31, 2000 letter were submitted in the Wellness petition. Studies that have been published since that letter were also included in the petitions. For purposes of this review, FDA, in determining the scientific support for a relationship between EPA and DHA omega-3 fatty acid dietary supplements and CHD, focused on the more recent studies to determine whether these studies added any support to the scientific evidence that was used for the current qualified health claim for EPA and DHA omega-3 fatty acid dietary supplements. For purposes of determining whether there is a relationship between EPA and DHA omega-3 fatty acids from conventional foods and reduced risk of CHD, FDA determined whether the relevant studies cited in the petition, in addition to other relevant studies that the agency had already reviewed in its previous reviews support a qualified health claim.

A. Assessment of the Intervention Studies

FDA identified a total of 10 intervention studies, not previously reviewed in 2000, for its current review of this qualified health claim (6 from the current petition[36]; 2 from the Wellness petition[37]; 1 from a comment[38]; 1 identified by FDA through a literature search[39]). FDA did not consider some of these studies in its current review for the following reasons: 1) Marchioli, et al. (2002) was a reanalysis of GISSI et al. (1999), which FDA reviewed in 2000, and provided no additional evidence relevant for establishing a substance-disease relationship; 2) Thies et al. (2003) and Maresta et al. (2002) measured outcomes (plaque stability and percutaneous transluminal coronary angioplasty (PTCA), respectively) that are not recognized as valid surrogate endpoints for CHD; 3) the studies by Ghafoorunissa et al. (2002), Laidlaw and Holub, et al. (2003) did not include control groups for EPA and DHA (Spilker, 1991); 4) Leng et al. (1998) did not include a control for gamma-linolenic acid (GLA), which constituted the majority of the treatment (approximately six times higher than EPA), thus there is no way to determine whether the effects were due to EPA; and 5) two intervention studies that reported no benefit on CHD incidence (Angerer et al., 2002; Nilsen et al., 2001) were conducted in CHD patients and the results could not be extrapolated to the general healthy population; therefore, these data were not considered relevant to FDA's review for establishing a substance-disease relationship in the general population. Thus, FDA considered only 2 intervention studies identified since the 2000 review as capable of supporting the substance/disease relationship (Finnegan et al., 2003; Woodman et al., 2002).

The studies by Finnegan et al. (2003) and Woodman et al. (2002) were randomized, placebo-controlled, double-blind[40] intervention studies that reported the effects of fish oil on blood pressure. Finnegan et al. (2003) reported the results from a study involving 150 moderately hyperlipidemic subjects[41] assigned to 1 of 5 interventions: fish oil (0.8 or 1.7 g/day

EPA+DHA); rapeseed and linseed oil (4.5 or 9.5 g/day ALA), or an n-6 PUFA control (sunflower and safflower oil) for 6 months. The fish oil intervention provided no benefit in CHD risk factors, including blood pressure, compared to the placebo control group. Woodman et al. (2002) was a 6-week intervention comparing EPA ethyl ester[42] (4 g/day) or DHA ethyl ester[42] (4 g/day) with olive oil (4 g/day) in type 2 diabetics[43] with hypertension (n=52). Neither EPA ethyl ester nor

DHA ethyl ester provided any benefit to blood pressure or any other CHD risk factor compared with the olive oil treated patients.

B. Assessment of the Observational Studies

FDA identified 10 observational studies not previously reviewed in 2000. These consisted of 6 prospective cohort studies (4 from the current petition[44]; 2 from the Wellness petition[45]), 3 nested case-control studies (2 from the current petition[46]; 1 from the Wellness petition[47]), and 1 ecological study from the current petition.[48]

Two of the 10 studies on fish consumption and CHD[49] were not considered in this review because these studies only reported total fish consumption without providing details of the fish type[50] or portion sizes, thus there is no way of knowing how much, if any, EPA and DHA omega-3 fatty acid was consumed. The remaining 8 observational studies[51] were of high to moderate quality. These observational studies provide only an estimated intake of EPA and DHA omega-3 fatty acids from fish consumption and provided only an association with disease risk, and not direct causality of disease risk.

Hu et al. (2002) reported results from the Nurses' Health Study, a prospective cohort study on female registered nurses (n=84,688) with a 16 year follow-up. Fish and omega-3 fatty acid intake were calculated as an average intake from all available dietary questionnaires up to the start of each 2-year follow-up interval in which events were reported. There was an inverse correlation observed between fish/omega-3 fatty acid consumption and incidence of CHD, including CHD deaths and nonfatal MI. A subgroup analysis of diabetic nurses from this cohort (n=5,103; Hu et al., 2003) observed a reduced risk of CHD from fish consumption but the association did not extend to estimated EPA and DHA omega-3 fatty acid consumption.

Albert et al. (2002) was a case-control study nested in the U.S. Physicians Health Study (Albert et al., 1998), which was considered in the 2000 review. The nested case-control study had a 17-year follow-up and reported a significant inverse relationship between whole blood omega-3 fatty acid concentrations and CHD death.

The study by Rissanen et al. (2000) reported 10-year follow-up results from the Kuopio Ischemic Heart Disease Risk Factor Study, which is an ongoing, prospective, population-based cohort study investigating risk factors for cardiovascular disease (CVD) and is part of the World Health Organization's (WHOs) MONICA project. The study enrolled 1,871 men who had no clinical CHD at baseline examination. The authors reported a decrease in acute coronary events in men at the highest quintile[52] of serum DHA+DPA[53] concentration compared with men at the lowest quintile.

Results from the Cardiovascular Health Study were reported by Mozaffarian et al. (2003). In this prospective cohort study, men (~1,500) and women (~2,400) aged ≥65 years were enrolled who were free of known CVD at baseline in 1989-1990 and had data on fish consumption. During the 9.3 years of follow-up, there were 247 ischemic heart disease (IHD)[54] deaths and 363 MIs. Estimated intake of EPA + DHA at baseline (0.55 g/day and 0.92 g/day) was associated with lower risk of fatal ischemic heart disease (IHD), but there was no association between EPA + DHA and non-fatal MI. This result is consistent with the report from a case-control study nested in the Cardiovascular Health Study (Lamaitre et al., 2003). A higher plasma concentration of EPA + DHA was associated with a lower risk of fatal IHD, but there was no association between plasma concentration of EPA + DHA and a risk of non-fatal IHD.

Hallgren et al. (2001) was a case-control study nested in the Västerbotten Intervention Programme, which was part of the WHOs MONICA project. In this study, 78 people (cases) developed an MI, and were matched against 156 controls subjects that were randomly selected from the study. Fish intake was assessed by a food frequency questionnaire (FFQ).[55] In addition, fatty acid composition of the plasma phospholipids, including EPA and DHA, was analyzed. There was no correlation between fish intake or blood EPA+DHA and acute MI.

Torres et al. (2000) compared fish consumption in Portuguese men living in a fishing village (n=50) or rural village (n=37) with IHD-related deaths based on death certificate records for the population. There was significantly more fish consumed in the fishing village compared with the rural village and this correlated with lower IHD deaths estimated from death certificate records for the two villages.

C. Other Data and Information

The Institute of Medicine (IOM) of the National Academy of Sciences has stated in its most recent Macronutrient Report that "Growing evidence suggests that dietary *n-3* polyunsaturated fatty acids (eicosapentaenoic acid

[EPA] and docosahexaenoic acid [DHA]) reduce the risk of coronary heart disease (CHD) and stroke."[56] Therefore, by concluding that there was only "growing evidence" that is "suggestive" of the relationship for this proposed claim, the IOM recognized limitations in the current data on omega-3 and its ability to reduce risk of CHD.

III. Strength of the Scientific Evidence

FDA relies primarily on human studies that are primary reports of data collection when attempting to establish a diet-disease relationship and has consistently identified two endpoints with which to identify disease risk reduction for purposes of health claims evaluations: a) reduction in incidence of the disease, and; b) beneficial changes in surrogate endpoints for the disease.[57] The most persuasive evidence for a relationship between EPA and DHA omega-3 fatty acids and reduced risk of CHD would be from intervention studies with EPA and DHA omega-3 fatty acids demonstrating reduced incidence of CHD in healthy populations (i.e., primary prevention). However, no such studies for EPA and DHA omega-3 fatty acids and CHD were identified. There were 2 small intervention studies in healthy populations that measured EPA and DHA effects on blood pressure, a CHD surrogate endpoint, but no benefit was observed in these studies. Thus, the scientific evidence from intervention studies available since the 2000 review with EPA and DHA omega-3 fatty acids as the test substance, did not show a relationship between omega-3 fatty acids and reduced risk of CHD in the general population.

The remaining studies considered were high to moderate quality observational studies on healthy populations. Of these, 3 studies (Albert et al., 1998, 2002; Hu et al., 2002; Mozaffarian et al., 2003 (also Lamaitre et al., 2003)) were conducted in populations relevant to the general U.S. population, across a broad age range (30 to 84 years) and consistently reported that EPA and DHA omega-3 fatty acids reduced the risk of CHD. The largest cohorts followed 84,688 women (Hu et al., 2002) and 20,551 men (Albert et al., 1998, 2002). Of the observational studies conducted in populations considered less relevant to the general U.S. population, 1 small study (n=78 cases) (Hallgren et al. 2001) reported no benefit; whereas 2 studies (Rissanan et al, 2000; Torres et al., 2000) with sample sizes of 1,871 and 50, respectively, reported an associated benefit. Observational studies provide less compelling evidence than intervention studies for a relationship between omega-3 fatty acids and reduced risk of CHD because they provide only an estimated intake of EPA and DHA omega-3 fatty acids rather than a direct measure. In addition, observational studies cannot separate the effect of EPA and DHA omega-3 fatty acids from the effects of other food components, and therefore it is not clear whether any purported benefit is related to the EPA and DHA omega-3 fatty acids or to other dietary factors. Observational studies provide only supportive rather than direct evidence for a relationship. For these reasons, FDA considers observational studies as less persuasive than intervention studies conducted in a general healthy population for establishing a substance-disease relationship. Nevertheless, primary prevention of CHD in healthy populations by EPA and DHA omega-3 fatty acids was observed in the majority of observational studies reviewed, which included 2 large prospective cohorts conducted in the US, the Nurses' Health Study (n=84,688; 16 year follow-up; Hu et al., 2002) and the U.S. Physicians Health Study (n=20,551; 11 to 17 year follow-up; Albert et al., 1998, 2002). In sum, the majority of observational studies consistently observed an associated CHD risk reduction from intake of EPA and DHA estimated from the diet in men and women in populations relevant (3 studies) or less relevant (2 studies) to the general U.S. population.

Given the inability of predicting CHD risk reduction in a general healthy population based on secondary prevention studies in diseased populations, and the limitations of the observational studies in separating the effects of EPA and DHA omega-3 fatty acids from other dietary factors, the agency evaluated other available evidence, as discussed in the October 31, 2000 letter, that provide support for a qualified health claim for EPA and DHA omega-3 fatty acids and reduced risk of CHD. As described in detail in the October 31,2000 letter,[58] FDA considered: (1) observational studies in the general healthy population in which fish consumption was the primary contributor of EPA and DHA omega-3 fatty acids, and (2) intervention studies in both the general healthy population and patients with established CHD that evaluated the effects of EPA and DHA omega-3 fatty acids on physiological endpoints (e.g., total cholesterol, LDL-cholesterol, HDL-cholesterol, VLDL-cholesterol, triglycerides, platelet aggregation), some of which have been proposed as possible mechanisms for the CHD risk reduction by EPA and DHA omega-3 fatty acids. Thus, FDA is not changing its position from that outlined in the October 31, 2000 letter on the EPA and DHA omega-3 fatty acid and CHD qualified claim that there is sufficient suggestive evidence that the benefit on CHD reported in CHD patients (i.e., secondary prevention) (reviewed in the October 31, 2000 letter) applies to the general population because of: (1) The primary CHD prevention in the general population associated with EPA and DHA consumption from fish in observational studies; and, (2) intervention studies demonstrating similar physiological effects of EPA and DHA in both the diseased and general populations. FDA still concludes that the weight of the scientific evidence for a health claim for EPA and DHA omega-3 fatty acids outweighs the scientific evidence against such a claim. The most significant change in the available body of evidence since 2000 is the additional observational studies, the majority of which consistently reported an associated benefit in CHD risk from EPA and DHA consumption from fish.

The observational studies estimating EPA and DHA omega-3 fatty acid intake from conventional foods support the expansion of the existing qualified health claim for EPA and DHA omega-3 fatty acids from dietary supplements and CHD to conventional foods. Therefore, FDA intends to consider the exercise of its enforcement discretion with regard to a qualified health claim on the label or in labeling of EPA and DHA omega-3 fatty acid-containing dietary supplements and conventional foods that provides a truthful and non-misleading description of the strength of the body of scientific evidence, e.g., "supportive but not conclusive research shows." Other factors that FDA intends to consider in deciding whether to exercise its enforcement discretion with regard to the use of this qualified health claim on particular foods, including dietary supplements, are discussed below.

IV. Other Enforcement Discretion Factors

Factors that FDA intends to consider in the exercise of its enforcement discretion for qualified health claims about EPA and DHA omega-3 fatty acids and reduced risk of coronary heart disease are discussed below. You should also know that FDA is considering its enforcement discretion as applying only to such foods in which EPA and DHA is an added ingredient that FDA has approved as a food additive or affirmed as GRAS or for which the agency has received a GRAS notification to which it did not object.

A. Total Fat, Saturated Fat, and Cholesterol Criteria for CHD-related Health Claims

In regulations authorizing CHD-related health claims, FDA has generally required, with a few exceptions, that foods bearing such claims meet the "low fat" criterion defined by 21 CFR 101.62(b)(2), the "low saturated fat" criterion defined by 21 CFR 101.62(c)(2), and the "low cholesterol" criterion defined by 21 CFR 101.62(d)(2) (see authorized claims in 21 CFR sections 101.75, 101.77, 101.81, 101.82, and 101.83). The agency discusses below how the agency intends to consider these criteria as factors in deciding whether to exercise its enforcement discretion for an omega-3 fatty acid qualified health claim on conventional foods and dietary supplements. Later in Section B, FDA discusses total fat, saturated fat, and cholesterol content disqualifying levels relative to the general requirement for health claims (21 CFR 101.14(a)(4)).

"Low Fat" Criterion

FDA has required in the past that foods bearing CHD health claims meet the requirement for "low fat" as defined by 21 CFR 101.62(b)(2). The requirement of the "low fat" criterion was first introduced in the dietary lipid and cardiovascular disease proposed rule (56 FR 60727 at 60739; November 27, 1991). FDA stated that, although total fat is not directly related to increased risk for CHD, it may have significant indirect effects. The agency stated that low fat diets facilitate reduction in the intake of saturated fat and cholesterol to recommended levels. Furthermore, the agency noted that obesity is a major risk factor for CHD, and dietary fats, which have more than twice as many calories per gram as proteins and carbohydrates, are major contributors to total calorie intakes. There have been several exceptions to this criterion in the past. Instead of the "low fat" criterion, fish and game meat are required to meet the "extra lean" criterion in the saturated fat and cholesterol and CHD health claim (21 CFR 101.75(c)(2)(ii)). Products derived from whole soybeans without added fat are exempted from the "low fat" criterion in the soy protein and CHD health claim (21 CFR 101.82(c)(2)(iii)(C)). In the plant sterol/stanol esters and CHD health claim, FDA does not require the "low fat" criterion but requires that total fat level of foods not exceed the total fat disqualifying level (21 CFR 101.14(a)(4)) with an exception for spread and dressing for salad on a per 50 g basis (21 CFR 101.83(c)(2)(iii)(C)). In not requiring the "low fat" criterion, FDA noted that the Dietary

Guidelines for Americans, 2000 (USDA & DHHS, 2000) recommended choosing a diet that is low in saturated fat and cholesterol and moderate in total fat. Specifically, the Dietary Guidelines recommended moderate amounts of foods high in unsaturated fat with a caution to avoid excess calories.

FDA concurs with the dietary guidelines that consuming diets low in saturated fat and cholesterol is more important in reducing CHD risk, than consuming diets low in total fat. Therefore, FDA has decided not to consider, as a factor in the exercise of its enforcement discretion, that either dietary supplements or conventional foods that bear an omega-3 fatty acid qualified health claim meet the "low fat" criterion.

"Low Saturated Fat" and "Low Cholesterol" Criteria

In regulations authorizing CHD health claims, FDA has also generally required that foods bearing the claims meet the "low saturated fat" criterion as defined by 21 CFR 101.62(c)(2), and the "low cholesterol" criterion as defined by 21 CFR 101.62(d)(2) (see authorized claims in 21 CFR sections 101.75, 101.77, 101.81, 101.82, and 101.83). FDA continues to believe that these criteria are important. Therefore, FDA intends to consider, as a factor in the exercise of its enforcement discretion, that conventional foods or dietary supplements that bear an omega-3 fatty acid qualified health claim meet the "low saturated fat" and "low cholesterol" criteria. However, there are some situations, as discussed below, when FDA does not believe that such a factor is important to a decision about the exercise of its enforcement discretion.

Low Saturated Fat

FDA intends to consider, as a factor in the exercise of its enforcement discretion, that individual foods other than fish that bear an omega-3 fatty acid qualified health claim, meet the "low saturated fat" criterion (21 CFR 101.62(c)(2)). This food category includes primarily foods enriched with EPA- and DHA-containing food ingredients. FDA intends to consider, as a factor in the exercise of its enforcement discretion for meal products as defined in 21 CFR 101.13(l) and main dishes as defined in 21 CFR 101.13(m) that such foods meet all criteria specified for the "low saturated fat" criteria (21 CFR 101.62(c)(2)). FDA believes that many foods would meet the "low saturated fat" criteria, as stated in the final rule for nutrient content claims (58 FR 2302 at 2339; January 6, 1993). The criteria, "no more than 15 percent of calories from saturated fat" for individual foods can be achieved due to calorie contribution from food ingredients other than fish oil in these foods. Later in this section, FDA defines fish as "products that are essentially all fish" and identifies nutrient content factors that it intends to consider in the exercise of its enforcement discretion for the qualified health claim.

FDA intends to exercise its enforcement discretion for EPA- and DHA-containing dietary supplements (whether softgels or liquid forms) that bear an omega-3 fatty acid qualified health claim, and that meet the low saturated fat criterion per reference amount customarily consumed (RACC). However, FDA does not intend to consider, as a factor in the exercise of its enforcement discretion, that "no more than 15 percent of calories be from saturated fat." In a fish oil, 20 - 30 percent of calories come from saturated fat (USDA National Nutrient Database for Standard Reference, Release 17). Because 100 percent fish oil dietary supplements usually have no other source of calories other than fish oil and reformulation is not possible to reduce percent of calories from saturated fat, fish oil dietary supplements would not be eligible for the qualified health claim if FDA decided to consider the 15 percent criterion in 21 CFR 101.62(c)(2) as a factor in the exercise of its enforcement discretion. FDA believes that not considering the 15 percent criterion as a factor in the exercise of its enforcement discretion is appropriate given that fish oils are derived from fish, which have been shown to be associated with a reduced risk of CHD in observational studies with healthy individuals. In the algal oil used in Martek's dietary supplements, 40 - 45 percent of the oil is DHA and 30 - 40 percent of calories come from saturated fat.[59] Because the algal oil is diluted by high oleic sunflower oil by 7 - 10 percent or by 50 - 60 percent to make the final DHA concentration specific to Martek's products (either 20 percent or 40 percent DHA), calorie contribution from saturated fat will be either a little less than 30 - 40 percent (for the 40 percent DHA product) or about 15 - 20 percent of calories (for the 20 percent DHA product). In the final oil, calories from saturated fat exceed 15 percent; however, the level overlaps with that of fish oils. Therefore, FDA intends to consider, as a factor in the exercise of its enforcement discretion, that dietary supplements that bear an omega-3 fatty acid qualified health claim meet the "equal to or less than 1 g of saturated fat per RACC" criterion in 21 CFR 101.62(c)(2) but does not intend to consider the "no more than 15 percent of calories from saturated fat" criterion as a factor in the exercise of its enforcement discretion.

Low Cholesterol

FDA intends to exercise enforcement discretion for an omega-3 fatty acid qualified health claim for individual foods, other than fish and dietary supplements, provided that such foods meet the low cholesterol criteria (21 CFR 101.62(d)(2)). The October 31, 2000 letter[60] and subsequent letters from FDA[61] [62] did not discuss the low cholesterol criteria for dietary supplements; however, most fish oil containing dietary supplements do not meet the low cholesterol criteria per 50 g. Most dietary supplements containing EPA and DHA omega-3 fatty acids (whether fish oils or algal oils) are in softgels, and the amount of these oils per RACC is very small. Serving sizes are usually in between 1 - 2 softgels. FDA estimates that 1 - 2 softgels may weigh about 1 - 3 g, containing about 0.5 - 2 g of fish oil or algal oil. This amount of fish oil would not exceed the "low cholesterol" criteria (20 mg) per RACC but would exceed the "low cholesterol" criteria per 50 g basis if the supplements contain 100 percent fish oil. Liquid forms of fish oil dietary supplements are much less common and provide usually one teaspoon as a serving size (containing 4.5 g of total fat). This amount of fish oil may contain about 22 - 34 mg of cholesterol (based upon USDA National Nutrient Database for Standard Reference, Release 17), but again such levels of consumption would not be common.

Algal oil dietary supplements are sold as softgels and the RACC of the supplement is one softgel, containing 0.5 g of the mixture of algal oil and high oleic sunflower oil.[63] Both the 100 mg DHA softgel and the 200 mg DHA softgel contain less than 2 mg of cholesterol, which is below the "low cholesterol" criteria (20 mg) per RACC. The cholesterol content of algal oil will vary. The algal oil that Martek proposed to use for various food categories in its GRAS notification (GRAS No. 000137) contains higher levels of cholesterol (about 380 mg/100g without dilution) than does the algal oil currently used for dietary supplements (about 30 mg/100g without dilution). Even if the algal oil with the high cholesterol content were used for dietary supplements, the cholesterol content per RACC would be very small (about 2 mg of cholesterol) because the amount of oil per serving (0.5 g) is small, but the cholesterol content would exceed the "low cholesterol" criteria (20 mg) per 50 g basis.

FDA estimates that 50 g of fish oils would contain about 240 to 380 mg of cholesterol (USDA National Nutrient Database for Standard Reference, Release 17). The algal oil currently used for dietary supplements (without the addition of sunflower oil) contains about 15 mg of cholesterol per 50 g.[64] The algal oil that Martek proposed to use for foods in its GRAS notification (GRAS No. 000137) (without the addition of sunflower oil) contains about 190 mg of cholesterol per 50 g.

Since it is highly unlikely that individuals would consume 50 g of dietary supplements containing EPA and DHA per day, FDA has decided that it is not necessary to consider, as a factor in the exercise of its enforcement discretion, that EPA- and DHA-containing dietary supplements weighing equal to or less than 5 g per RACC contain no more than 20 mg of cholesterol on a 50 g basis. However, FDA has decided that it is necessary to consider, as a factor in the exercise of its enforcement discretion, that EPA- and DHA-containing dietary supplements that weigh more than 5 g per RACC contain no more than 20 mg of cholesterol on a 50 g basis.

"Extra Lean" Criterion for Fish

FDA has defined fish in 21 CFR 123.3(d) as "fresh or saltwater finfish, crustaceans, other forms of aquatic animal life (including, but not limited to, alligator, frog, aquatic turtle, jellyfish, sea cucumber, and sea urchin and the roe of such animals) other than birds or mammals, and all mollusks, where such animal life is intended for human consumption." For the purpose of omega-3 fatty acid qualified health claims about fish, FDA intends to consider certain factors in the exercise of its enforcement discretion for use of these claims on "products that are essentially all fish." This category includes fish without any added ingredients and fish with a small amount of added fat or carbohydrate that meets the definition of an insignificant amount in 21 CFR 101.9(f)(1). Examples of "products that are essentially all fish" are raw fish, boiled fish, and broiled fish.

In the past, fish was given an exception for the "low saturated fat" criterion and "the low cholesterol" criterion, along with game meat, in the health claim about diets low in saturated fat and cholesterol and reduced risk of CHD (21 CFR 101.75 (c)(2)(ii)). Instead of the "low saturated fat and low cholesterol" criteria, fish was required to meet the "extra lean" criterion as defined in 21 CFR 101.62(e)(3) (i.e, contains less than 5 g total fat, less than 2 g saturated fat, and less than 95 mg cholesterol per reference amount customarily consumed and per 100 g.).

In applying the "extra lean" criterion to fish, FDA was not thinking about oily fish that are rich in EPA and DHA omega-3 fatty acids. Most fish that are a rich source of EPA and DHA exceed the "extra lean" criterion for saturated fat (2 g of saturated fat per RACC) but do not exceed the saturated fat disqualifying level (4 g of saturated fat per RACC). One of the ways that FDA determines whether to consider nutrient content eligibility criteria as a factor in the exercise of its enforcement discretion is whether there are risk reduction data among healthy individuals that would suggest that there may be a benefit from consumption of the food, even though the food does not meet the nutrient content eligibility criteria. Such data, for purposes of this review, would include an association with a lower risk of CHD, shown in observational studies conducted in apparently healthy individuals. Because the following observational studies: Albert et al., 1998, 2002; Hu et al., 2002; Mozaffarian et al., 2003 showed an association of fish intake with reduced risk of CHD in apparently healthy individuals, FDA has decided that the agency does not need to consider, as a factor in the exercise of its enforcement discretion for products that are essentially all fish, that such products meet the "extra lean" criterion for saturated fat. However, FDA has decided to consider, as a factor in the exercise of its enforcement discretion for products that are essentially all fish, that such products meet the "extra lean" criterion for cholesterol (95 mg of cholesterol per RACC). Most fish that are rich sources of EPA and DHA do not exceed the "extra lean" criterion for cholesterol; thus, this approach should not disqualify many products that are essentially all fish. As discussed earlier, FDA now considers the "low fat" criterion not important here; therefore, FDA is not considering the "extra lean" criterion for total fat, as a factor in exercising its enforcement discretion, which is not very different from how the agency approached its consideration of the "low fat" criteria as a factor for products that are essentially all fish.

B. Disqualifying Nutrient Levels

Under the general requirements for health claims (21 CFR 101.14(e)(3)) a food may not bear a health claim if that food exceeds any of the disqualifying nutrient levels for total fat, saturated fat, cholesterol, or sodium established in § 101.14(a)(4). Section 101.14 applies to all health claims regardless of types of diseases and health-related conditions. The disqualifying nutrient levels vary for individual foods, meal products, and main dishes. Disqualifying total fat levels are above 13.0 g per RACC, per label serving size and per 50 g if the RACC is 30 g or less or 2 tablespoons or less for individual foods, above 26.0 g per label serving size for meal products, and above 19.5 g per label serving size for main dish products. Disqualifying saturated fat levels are above 4.0 g per RACC, per label serving size and per 50 g if the RACC is 30 g or less or 2 tablespoons or less for individual foods, above 8.0 g per label serving size for meal products, and above 6.0 g per label serving size for main dish products. Disqualifying cholesterol levels are

above 60 mg per RACC, per label serving size and per 50 g if the RACC is 30 g or less or 2 tablespoons or less for individual foods, above 120 mg per label serving size for meal products, and above 90 mg per label serving size for main dish products. Disqualifying sodium levels are 480 mg per RACC, per label serving size and per 50 g if the RACC is 30 g or less or 2 tablespoons or less for individual foods, above 960 mg per label serving size for meal products, and above 720 mg per label serving size for main dish products.

The general requirements for health claims also provide for FDA to authorize a health claim for food despite the fact that a nutrient in the food exceeds the disqualifying level, if the agency finds that such a claim will assist consumers in maintaining healthy dietary practices. In such cases, the label must also bear a disclosure statement that complies with 21 CFR

101.13(h), highlighting the nutrient that exceeds the disqualifying level (21 CFR 101.14(e)(3)).

The application of these regulatory provisions to omega-3 fatty acid qualified health claims on dietary supplements and conventional foods is discussed below.

"Total Fat" Disqualifying Level

In the previous section (Section IV A), FDA explained that the agency has decided not to consider, as a factor in the exercise of its enforcement discretion, that dietary supplements and conventional foods that bear an omega-3 fatty acid qualified health claim meet the "low fat" criterion as defined by 21 CFR 101.62(b)(2). FDA notes that there is a large difference in the amount of total fat between the "low fat" criterion and the disqualifying total fat level. For example, the "low fat" criterion for individual foods is equal to or less than 3 g per RACC and per 50 g if RACC is 30 g or less or 2 tablespoons or less. The total fat disqualifying level for individual foods is above 13 g per RACC, per label serving size and per 50 g if RACC is 30 g or less or 2 tablespoon or less. Thus, there is a difference of 10 g for individual foods between the "low fat" criterion and the total fat disqualifying level. In addition, the disqualifying levels of nutrients are a required element of all health claims (i.e., cancer claims, osteoporosis claims, CHD claims) under 21 CFR 101.14. Because FDA has not evaluated the implications of eliminating the total fat disqualifying level for all possible health claims, FDA believes that it would be appropriate to consider, as a factor in the exercise of its enforcement discretion that conventional foods and dietary supplements that bear an omega-3 fatty acid qualified claim meet the total fat disqualifying level. However, there are some situations, as discussed below, when FDA does not believe that such a factor is important to a decision about the exercise of its enforcement discretion.

Products that are Essentially all Fish

Based upon the data the agency has (USDA National Nutrient Database for Standard Reference, Release 17), FDA believes that total fat content of almost all fish that are a rich source of EPA and DHA are below the total fat disqualifying level (13.0 g of total fat per RACC). A few fish including halibut, herring, and mackerel contain total fat exceeding 13 g but contain less than 16.0 g of total fat per RACC. Because the observational studies that showed an association of fish intake with reduced risk of CHD do not distinguish fish species, FDA has no basis to discriminate one type of fish from any other type. In addition, the amount of total fat exceeding the disqualifying total fat level by these fish is small (about 3 g); therefore, FDA has decided to consider, as a factor in the exercise of its enforcement discretion, that products that are essentially all fish not exceed a total fat content per RACC of 16.0 g. If the total fat level of products that are essentially all fish exceeds the disqualifying level as defined by 21 CFR 101.14(a)(4), the disclosure statement (i.e., "See nutrition information for total fat, saturated fat, and cholesterol content") required by §101.14(e)(3) must be placed immediately adjacent to and directly beneath the claim, with no intervening material, in the same size, typeface, and contrast as the claim itself. Under 21 CFR 101.9(j)(10), if raw fish bears a health claim, nutrition labeling of the fish must be presented to the public in accordance with 21 CFR 101.45. Nutrition labeling of fish other than raw fish must follow the regulations specified in 21 CFR 101.9.

Other Conventional Foods and Dietary Supplements

Unlike fish, other EPA- and DHA-containing conventional foods that contain high levels of total fat have not been shown to have an association with a reduced risk of CHD in a population free of CHD. Therefore, FDA intends to consider the "total fat" disqualifying levels as defined in 21 CFR 101.14(a)(4) for all conventional foods, other than products that are essentially all fish, in the agency's consideration for the exercise of enforcement discretion for the omega-3 qualified health claim.

A comment suggested that FDA apply 6.5 g or less of total fat per RACC and per labeled serving instead of the "low fat" criterion as an eligibility criterion for spreads and mayonnaise-type dressings and requested an exemption for these foods from the "low fat" criterion and the total fat disqualifying level per 50 g. As explained earlier in this letter (Section IV A), FDA does not intend to consider the "low fat" criterion as a factor in the exercise of its enforcement discretion for the omega-3 qualified health claim. The 50 g weight-based criterion was developed, in part, to deal with foods with small serving sizes (e.g., foods with 15-30 g RACCs) that are dense in nutrients such as fat or sodium. As the agency noted in the final rule for general requirements for health claims, foods with small serving sizes may be consumed more frequently than once a day (58 FR 2478 at 2496; January 6, 1993). Health claims on foods such as spreads (RACC is 15 g) and mayonnaise-type dressings (RACC is 15 g) would promote their consumption, and could contribute to large intakes of total fat and calories that might not help to maintain healthy dietary practices. In addition, the level of scientific evidence linking EPA and DHA omega-3 fatty acids to reduced risk of CHD does not reach the significant scientific evidence standard; therefore, there is a fair amount of uncertainty as to whether frequent consumption of EPA and DHA enriched spreads and mayonnaise-type dressings that contribute a large amount of total fat and calories would maintain healthy dietary practices, compared to other foods that do not contain such high amounts of fats and calories in such small serving sizes. Also, there are many foods that are naturally lower in total fat on a weight basis than spreads and mayonnaise-type dressings to which EPA and DHA containing food ingredients could be added; therefore, consumers would have many foods to choose from to obtain the purported health benefit of EPA and DHA. Therefore, FDA has decided to not accept the comment's suggestion, and instead, considers compliance with the "total fat" disqualifying levels as a condition of its enforcement discretion for spreads and mayonnaise-type dressings.

However, FDA does believe that it would be appropriate to consider, as a factor in the exercise of its enforcement discretion, that dietary supplements that weigh equal to or less than 5 g per RACC that exceed the per 50 g total fat disqualifying level (i.e., above 13.0 g of total fat per 50 g), be eligible to bear an omega-3 fatty acid qualified health claim. As explained earlier, most EPA- and DHA-containing dietary supplements are in softgel forms. A serving of fish oil or algal oil dietary supplements in softgels normally contain extremely small amount of total fat (about 0.5 - 2 g of total fat). Liquid forms of fish oils are rare and the serving size is labeled as a teaspoonful. A teaspoonful of fish oil contains about 4.5 g of total fat. FDA is not aware of algal oil dietary supplements in a liquid form. In either softgel or liquid forms, one serving of an EPA- and DHA-containing dietary supplement that weighs equal to or less than 5 g per RACC would provide a very small amount of total fat. It is highly unlikely that individuals would consume 50 g of dietary supplements per day. Therefore, FDA believes that it would be appropriate to consider the exercise of its enforcement discretion for the use of an omega-3 fatty acid qualified health claim for dietary supplements that weigh equal to or less than 5 g per RACC but that exceed the disqualifying level for total fat per 50 g. If the total fat level of dietary supplements that weigh equal to or less than 5 g per RACC exceeds the per 50 g disqualifying level, the disclosure statement (i.e., "See nutrition information for total fat content") required by 21 CFR 101.14(e)(3) must be placed immediately adjacent to and directly beneath the claim, with no intervening material, in the same size, typeface, and contrast as the claim itself. FDA does not intend to exercise its enforcement discretion with respect to all other applicable labeling requirements that apply to dietary supplements, including 21 CFR 101.36(b)(2) that requires dietary supplements to declare the amount of nutrients when the level exceeds the amount that can be declared as zero. Please note that dietary supplements that are not subject to FDA's enforcement discretion that weigh more than 5 g per RACC are subject to the per 50 g total fat disqualifying level, consistent with 21 CFR 101.14(a)(4).

"Saturated Fat" Disqualifying Level

In exercising enforcement discretion for the omega-3 qualified health claim, FDA intends to consider, as a factor in the exercise of its enforcement discretion, the disqualifying saturated fat level, as defined in 21 CFR 101.14(a)(4), for all conventional foods including products that are essentially all fish. FDA believes that almost all products that are essentially all fish do not exceed the saturated fat disqualifying level. FDA also believes that many other conventional foods to which EPA and DHA could be added do not exceed the saturated fat disqualifying level.

The EPA- and DHA-containing dietary supplements generally exceed the saturated fat disqualifying level per 50 g (i.e., above 4.0 g of saturated fat per 50 g). Fish oils contain 10 - 15 g of saturated fat per 50 g (USDA National Nutrient Database for Standard Reference, Release 17). The algal oil used for dietary supplements contains 15 - 20 g of saturated fat per 50 g.[65] A serving of EPA- and DHA- containing dietary supplements in softgels normally contain about 0.5 - 2 g of total fat. This amount of fish oil or algal oil does not contain more than 1 g of saturated fat. Also, a teaspoon of fish oil contains about 0.9 - 1.4 g of saturated fat, a level that is below the saturated fat disqualifying level per RACC (4 g). Given that the suggested consumption level is so low, it is highly unlikely that individuals would consume 50 g of dietary supplements, which might contain about 10 - 20 g of saturated fat. Because the amount of saturated fat consumed through dietary supplements which weigh equal to or less than 5 g per RACC is small, FDA has decided not to consider, as a factor in the exercise of its enforcement discretion, that such dietary supplements bearing an omega-3 fatty acid qualified health claim meet the per 50 g saturated fat disqualifying level. If the saturated fat level of dietary supplements that weigh equal to or less than 5 g per RACC exceeds the per 50 g disqualifying level, the disclosure statement (i.e., "See nutrition information for saturated fat content") required by §101.14(e)(3) must be placed immediately adjacent to and directly beneath the claim, with no intervening material, in the same size, typeface, and contrast as the claim itself. Dietary supplements that weigh more than 5 g per RACC must comply with the per 50 g saturated fat disqualifying level, consistent with 21 CFR 101.14(a)(4).

"Cholesterol" Disqualifying Level

Products that are Essentially all Fish

As discussed earlier, FDA applies the "extra lean" criterion for cholesterol as a factor in the exercise of its enforcement discretion for the omega-3 fatty acid qualified health claim. The "extra lean" criterion allows more cholesterol per RACC (95 mg per RACC) than does the cholesterol disqualifying level (60 mg per RACC) for products that are essentially all fish. The agency has decided not to consider, as a factor in the exercise of its enforcement discretion, that these products bearing an omega-3 fatty acid qualified health claim meet the cholesterol disqualifying level because, as discussed earlier, observational studies (Albert et al., 1998, 2002; Hu et al., 2002; Mozaffarian et al., 2003) conducted among healthy individuals showed an association of fish intake with reduced risk of CHD. If the cholesterol level of products that are essentially all fish exceed the cholesterol disqualifying level, the disclosure statement (i.e., "See nutrition information for cholesterol content") required by §101.14(e)(3) must be placed immediately adjacent to and directly beneath the claim, with no intervening material, in the same size, typeface, and contrast as the claim itself.

Other Conventional Foods and Dietary Supplements

FDA intends to consider, as a factor in the exercise of its enforcement discretion, the disqualifying cholesterol level, as defined in 21 CFR 101.14(a)(4), for all conventional foods other than products that are essentially all fish and dietary supplements. FDA does not intend to consider, as a factor in the exercise of its enforcement discretion, that dietary supplements weighing equal to or less than 5 g per RACC that bear an omega-3 fatty acid qualified health claim meet the cholesterol disqualifying criteria on a per 50 g basis for the same reasons discussed in the "low cholesterol" criteria in section IV A. If the cholesterol level of dietary supplements that weigh equal to or less than 5 g per RACC exceeds the per 50 g disqualifying level, the disclosure statement (i.e., "See nutrition information for cholesterol content") required by §101.14(e)(3) must be placed immediately adjacent to and directly beneath the claim, with no intervening material, in the same size, typeface, and contrast as the claim itself. Dietary supplements that weigh more than 5 g per RACC must comply with the per 50 g cholesterol disqualifying level, consistent with 21 CFR 101.14(a)(4).

"Sodium" Disqualifying Level

FDA intends to consider, as a factor in the exercise of its enforcement discretion for the use of an omega-3 fatty acid qualified health claim, the sodium disqualifying nutrient level as specified in 21 CFR 101.14(a)(4) for dietary supplements and conventional foods, including products that are essentially all fish.

C. 10 Percent Minimum Nutrient Content Requirement

Under the general requirements for health claims, a conventional food may not bear a health claim unless it contains, prior to any nutrient addition, at least 10 percent of the Daily Value for vitamin A, vitamin C, iron, calcium, protein, or dietary fiber per RACC (see 21 CFR 101.14(e)(6)). The purpose of this provision is to prevent the use of health claims on foods of minimal nutritional value.

Dietary Supplements

The 10 percent minimum nutrient content requirement does not apply to dietary supplements (21 CFR 101.14(e)(6)).

"Products that are Essentially all Fish"

The 10% minimum nutrient content requirement per RACC for protein is 5 grams. Products that are essentially all fish contain more than 5 grams of protein per RACC. Thus, FDA believes that such products would qualify for the requirement. FDA intends to consider, as a factor in the exercise of its enforcement discretion, that products that are essentially all fish that bear an omega-3 fatty acid qualified health claim meet the 10 percent minimum nutrient content requirement.

Other Conventional Foods

FDA intends to consider, as a factor in the exercise of its enforcement discretion, that other conventional foods meet the 10 percent minimum nutrient content requirement. A comment requested that FDA eliminate the minimum nutrient content requirement for dressings for salad and mayonnaise-type dressings. These foods are almost completely devoid of the nutrients that are required to be present at 10 percent or more of reference daily intake as specified in 21 CFR 101.14(e)(6). These foods are the type of foods that FDA had in mind when it required the 10 percent minimum nutrient content as a general requirement for health claims because nutritional values are low while fat and calories are high. FDA considers that the presence of an omega-3 qualified health claim on salad dressings and mayonnaise-type dressings that do not meet the 10% minimum nutrient content requirement would be inconsistent with the principle of health claims, i.e., that health claims should be used on foods that help maintain healthy dietary practices. Since there are many conventional foods enriched with EPA and DHA omega-3 fatty acids that could meet the 10 percent minimum nutrient content requirement, FDA believes that there is no need to consider enforcement discretion for a qualified claim on dressings for salad and mayonnaise-type dressings that do not meet the 10 percent minimum nutrient content requirement.

D. Context of a Total Daily Diet

A provision of the general requirements for health claims requires that a health claim enable the public to comprehend the information provided and to understand the relative significance of such information in the context of the total daily diet (see section 403(r)(3)(B)(iii) of the Act (21 U.S.C. 343 (r)(3)(B)(iii) and 21 CFR 101.14(d)(2)(v))). For health claims pertaining to coronary heart disease that are authorized by regulation (e.g., health claims about fruit, vegetables and grain products that contain fiber, particularly soluble fiber, and risk of coronary heart disease (21 CFR 101.77)), FDA requires information relative to a total diet low in saturated fat and cholesterol because this is an essential part of dietary guidance for reducing the risk of CHD.

However, in FDA's previous letter, regarding omega-3 fatty acids and CHD qualified health claims (February 8, 2002 letter[66]), the agency decided that its exercise of enforcement discretion was not contingent on the use of the sentence (i.e., "It is known that diets low in saturated fat and cholesterol may reduce the risk of heart disease.") in connection with the claim. FDA made this decision because the scientific data that the agency relied on did not specifically evaluate whether the potential benefit of consuming EPA and DHA omega-3 fatty acids on CHD risk depends upon subjects consuming diets low in saturated fat and cholesterol. Because FDA is not aware of any new scientific data that might shed light on this subject, the agency has decided to take the same position discussed in the February 8, 2002 letter. Thus, FDA will not consider the exercise of its enforcement discretion to be contingent upon the use of the phrase or sentence relating diets low in saturated fat and cholesterol in the claim.

E. Daily Dietary Intake Needed to Achieve the Claimed Effect

The general requirements for health claims provide that, if the claim is about the effects of consuming the substance at other than decreased dietary levels, the level of the substance must be sufficiently high and in an appropriate form to justify the claim. Where no definition for "high" has been established, the claim must specify the daily dietary intake necessary to achieve the claimed effect (see 21 CFR 101.14(d)(2)(vii)). Several comments stated that 0.5 to 1 g of EPA and DHA are the effective daily dietary intake levels of EPA and DHA in reducing the risk of CHD, and that about one fourth of the amount (100 to 250 mg of EPA and DHA) should be the minimum level of EPA and DHA per RACC necessary to bear the qualified health claim. One comment suggested 32 mg of EPA and DHA as the minimum level of EPA and DHA necessary to bear the qualified health claim.

The minimum daily dietary intake level is based on the total amount of substance consumed in a day (g/day) and is calculated by summing the amount consumed through supplementation with the amount consumed in the diet. However, as concluded in FDA's previous review on omega-3 fatty acids and CHD (October 31, 2000 letter[67]), the agency finds that this provision cannot be applied to the qualified claim for EPA and DHA omega-3 fatty acids and reduced risk of CHD because the scientific evidence for this relationship is not conclusive and does not support the establishment of a recommended daily dietary intake level or even a possible level of effect for the general U.S. population. Therefore, the agency continues to consider any label or labeling suggesting a level of omega-3 fatty acids to be useful in achieving a reduction in the risk of CHD for the general healthy population to be false and misleading under Section 403(a) of the Act.

FDA concludes that the use of EPA and DHA omega-3 fatty acids as dietary supplements and as an ingredient in conventional foods is safe and lawful under 21 CFR 101.14, provided that the daily intakes of EPA and DHA omega-3 fatty acids do not exceed 3 grams per person per day from conventional foods and dietary supplement sources. Further, in order to help ensure that a consumer does not exceed an intake of 3 grams per person per day of EPA and DHA omega-3 fatty acids from consumption of a dietary supplement with the qualified health claim, FDA intends to consider, as a factor in the exercise of its enforcement discretion, that an EPA- and DHA-containing dietary supplement bearing a qualified claim not recommend or suggest in its labeling a daily intake exceeding 2 grams of EPA and DHA.

As previously stated, the agency is encouraging manufacturers to limit the products that bear the qualified health claim for omega-3 fatty acids and reduced risk of CHD to a daily intake of 1 gram. Further, the agency would consider dietary supplements that bear the qualified claim that encourage intakes (in labeling or under ordinary conditions of use) above 2 grams per day to be outside the scope of the agency's consideration of its enforcement discretion. FDA expects EPA and DHA levels of conventional foods enriched with EPA and DHA containing food ingredients not to exceed the maximum use level specified in the menhaden oil GRAS affirmation or the GRAS notifications (to which FDA did not object) specific to their oil and food category. Also, as explained in the section on safety of foods containing EPA and DHA (see section I.C.), FDA intends to consider, as a factor in the exercise of its enforcement discretion, that conventional foods and dietary supplements that bear an omega-3 fatty acid qualified health claim declare the amount of EPA and DHA per serving in the claim.

V. Fish and Mercury

FDA received a few comments specific to the safety of fish and fish oils. The Martek petition stated that the presence of mercury in fish can harm the developing nervous systems of unborn children, infants, and young children, and therefore, the presence of mercury in fish and fish derivatives needs to be addressed in the health claim. The Martek petition referenced the March 2004 FDA advisory that cautions pregnant women, women who might become pregnant, nursing mothers and young children against the consumption of certain fish, and that suggests limits to weekly intake of other fish and shellfish. Specifically, the Martek petition stated that certain fish (including shark, swordfish, king mackerel, and tile fish) and other fish that similarly become included in a future FDA advisory should be ineligible to bear the proposed health claim. The Martek petition further suggested that when the health claim appears on other fish, it should be accompanied by an advisory statement suggesting a limited weekly intake for a vulnerable population of pregnant women, women of childbearing age, nursing mothers, and young children. In addition, the Martek petition stated that sources of omega-3 fatty acids derived from fish (such as fish oils) should be ineligible for the health claim unless the oil has been tested and found to contain less than 0.025 ppm of mercury. Finally, the Martek petition stated that the presence of mercury may offset the cardio-protective effects of omega-3 fatty acids, and therefore, that the claim would be misleading if it appeared on fish that contained elevated levels of mercury. The Martek petition stated that the mercury specific limitations and the advisory language would be needed to ensure that the claim is truthful and not misleading under sections 403(a) and 201(n) of the Act.

In a comment that Mr. Emord submitted in response to the Martek petition, Mr. Emord concurred with the suggested prohibition of the use of the proposed health claim on shark, king mackerel, swordfish, and tile fish and with the need for an advisory as part of the claim on other fish, but only for those fish that contained 1 ppm total mercury or less. Mr. Emord disagreed with the Martek petition that mercury may diminish the protective effects of omega-3 fatty acids on heart health. Finally, Mr. Emord presented modified language for the proposed advisory statement on other fish and provided a statement for use on omega-3 fatty acid dietary supplements, containing 1 ppm total mercury or less, stating that intake of omega-3 fatty acids from such supplements should be limited to no more than 3000 mg/day. Mr. Emord suggested setting 1 ppm mercury as an eligibility criterion for qualified health claims for all foods and dietary supplements.

Yet another comment asserted that most of the refining techniques ensure the removal of contaminants, such as mercury, from fish oil products, and often achieve levels below the level of detection. The comment asserted that highly refined fish oils are safe to ingest at the recommended levels when consumed as conventional foods or as dietary supplements. FDA is not aware of any contrary information.

However, FDA does question the basis of the Martek petition's assertion that in order to bear omega-3 fatty acid qualified health claims, fish oils have to be tested and confirmed to contain less than 0.025 ppm of mercury, a level the Martek petition claims is the limit of detection for the most sensitive test accepted as standard by the Association of Official Analytical Chemists. Top selling fish oil dietary supplements have been reported not to contain any significant amount of mercury (Foran et al., 2003 and Consumer Reports, 2003) and FDA is not aware of any data that has shown otherwise. Further, FDA notes that in order for conventional foods to bear omega-3 fatty acid qualified health claims, EPA- and DHA-containing food ingredients have to be generally recognized as safe (GRAS). The determination of GRAS includes an evaluation of possible contaminants including mercury. For instance, the menhaden oil GRAS affirmation (21 CFR 185.1472(a)(2)(ix)) sets a limit on mercury content (0.5 ppm) and GRAS notifications for other EPA and DHA containing food ingredients[68] did not raise FDA's concerns for mercury. Given that there are no data showing that the mercury content of fish oils are high and that the

Martek petition's reason for setting 0.025 ppm was based upon detection limit rather than effect on health, FDA is not persuaded to adopt the Martek petition's request.

With regard to Mr. Emord's comment suggesting setting 1 ppm as an eligibility criterion for conventional foods and dietary supplements, as mentioned previously, FDA does not expect that the mercury content of dietary supplements would be close to 1 ppm. Also, the GRAS notification process for conventional foods ensures that the mercury level specifications for EPA and DHA containing food ingredients are low enough to protect the public health. Therefore, FDA concludes that there is no need for the agency's exercise of enforcement discretion for the omega-3 fatty acid qualified health claim on fish oils to be contingent on additional specifications for mercury.

FDA disagrees with the petitioners' contention that the omega-3 fatty acid qualified health claim should be accompanied by a product label statement about mercury content of fish and possible harmful health effects to the vulnerable population of pregnant women, women who might become pregnant, nursing mothers, and young children. For some time, FDA has been addressing the issue of reducing the exposure to the harmful effects of mercury by communicating with this target population (pregnant women, women who might become pregnant, nursing mothers, and parents of young children) through the use of consumer advisories. The latest consumer advisory was issued in March 2004 jointly by FDA and the Environmental Protection Agency.[69] This advisory includes information about mercury and makes recommendations about the kinds and amount of fish to eat and to avoid.

Agencies are granted broad discretion in determining the means by which to pursue policy goals.[70] Furthermore, the agency believes that the consumer advisory is a preferable method to educate the target population about mercury in fish, for several reasons. First, consumer advisories are communicated to the target population directly.[71] Second, FDA believes that the advisory approach is more effective than a product label statement in relaying the complex messages about mercury in fish and shellfish. For example, the current advisory distinguishes the mercury content in the fish by identifying specifically which fish to eat and not eat and how much fish to eat of the different types. The advisory also identifies which common fish are low in mercury. This level of clarity and detail would be difficult to provide on a product label statement, due to the limited space. Furthermore, confusion could take place when different kinds of label statements are put on different species of commercial fish and not on locally caught fish. Third, a label statement that reaches the public at large can also have unintended adverse public health consequences. FDA focus group results suggest that people who are not in the target audience (i.e., women who are not nursing and not likely to become pregnant, and men) might eat less fish or refrain from eating fish altogether when they receive information about the mercury content of fish and possible harmful health effects to pregnant women, women who might become pregnant, nursing mothers, and young children (ORC Macro, 2003). Therefore, the statement about possible harmful effects of mercury accompanying the qualified health claim would likely have the effect of negating the qualified health claim. In summary, FDA has decided that it is preferable not to use a label statement about mercury and possible harmful effect to pregnant women, women who might become pregnant, nursing mothers and young children as a condition for the agency's enforcement discretion for the omega-3 fatty acid qualified health claims.

FDA also disagrees with petitioners' suggestion that FDA not allow the use of omega-3 fatty acid qualified health claims on the four fish the FDA advisory warns the target population not to consume. FDA has not issued any advice about the consumption of these fish for the general public, particularly the non-target population (i.e., men, adolescents, women who are not nursing and not likely to become pregnant) and the agency does not believe that it is necessary to prohibit labels of these fish from bearing omega-3 fatty acid qualified health claims.

Finally, FDA disagrees with the assertion in the Martek petition that it would be misleading not to have a statement about mercury's effects on the cardio-protective effects of EPA and DHA omega-3 fatty acids from fish. There are only a few studies on this subject and results are inconsistent. A case-control study by Guallar et al. (2002) showed an association between mercury levels in toenails and increased risk of myocardial infarction. A case-control study within a large prospective cohort, conducted by Yoshizawa et al. (2003) found no association between mercury levels in toenails and CHD risk. After excluding dentists, who were found to have higher levels of mercury in toenails than other study participants, the analysis did not find a significant association between mercury levels in toenails and CHD risk. A cohort study by Salonen et al. (1995) did find an association between mercury levels in hair and increased risk of acute myocardial infarction. But, a case-control study within an ongoing community intervention program on cardiovascular disease and diabetes prevention, conducted by Hallgren et al. (2001), found an association between the concentration of mercury in erythrocytes and decreased risk of CHD. Thus, these observational studies showed inconsistent results regarding the relationship between mercury and CHD. FDA believes that whether mercury has any role in CHD risk is an unanswered scientific question. Consequently, it is not possible to determine whether mercury counteracts the cardio-protective effects of EPA and DHA omega-3 fatty acids from fish. In summary, FDA finds that the Martek assertion that mercury can counteract the beneficial effect of omega-3 fatty acids as speculative, and FDA will not consider, as a factor in the exercise of its enforcement discretion, that foods that bear an omega-3 fatty acid qualified health claim also bear the suggested label statement, "At high levels, mercury may diminish the protective effects of omega-3 fatty acids on heart health."

VI. Conclusions

Based on FDA's consideration of the scientific evidence and other information submitted with your petition, and other pertinent scientific evidence and information, FDA concludes that there is sufficient evidence for a qualified health claim, provided that the qualified claim is appropriately worded so as to not mislead consumers. Thus, FDA will consider exercising enforcement discretion for the following qualified health claim:

> Supportive but not conclusive research shows that consumption of EPA and DHA omega-3 fatty acids may reduce the risk of coronary heart disease. One serving of [Name of the food] provides [ ] gram of EPA and DHA omega-3 fatty acids. [See nutrition information for total fat, saturated fat, and cholesterol content.]

Dietary supplements may declare the amount of EPA and DHA per serving in "Supplement Facts," instead of making the declaration in the claim.

FDA intends to consider exercising enforcement discretion for the above qualified claim when all other factors for enforcement discretion identified in Section IV of this letter are met.

Please note that scientific information is subject to change, as are consumer consumption patterns. FDA intends to evaluate new information that becomes available to determine whether it necessitates a change in this decision. For example, scientific evidence may become available that will support significant scientific agreement or that will no longer support the use of a qualified claim, or that may raise safety concerns about the substance that is the subject of the claim.

Sincerely,
William K. Hubbard
Associate Commissioner for Policy and Planning

REFERENCES

Albert, C.M., C.H. Hennekens, C.J. O'Donnell, U.A. Ajani, V.J. Carey, W.C. Willett., J.N. Ruskin, and J.E. Manson. Fish consumption and risk of sudden cardiac death. *Journal of the American Medical Association.* 1998; 279(1):23-28.

Albert, C.M., H. Campos, M.J. Stampfer, P.M. Ridker, J.E. Manson., W.C. Willett, and J. Ma. Blood levels of long-chain n-3 fatty acids and the risk of sudden death. *The New England Journal of Medicine.* 2002; 346(15):1113-1118.

Angerer, P., W. Kothny, S. Störk, and C. von Schacky. Effect of dietary supplementation with ω-3 fatty acids on progression of atherosclerosis in carotid arteries. *Cardiovascular Research.* 2002; 54(1):183-190.

Ascherio, A. Epidemiologic studies on dietary fats and coronary heart disease. *American Journal of Medicine.* 2002;113 Suppl 9B:9S-12S.

Baylin, A., E.K. Kabagambe, A. Ascherio, D. Spiegelman, and H. Campos. Adipose tissue α-linolenic acid and nonfatal acute myocardial infarction in Costa Rica. *Circulation.* 2003;107(12):1586-1591.

Bemelmans, W.J., J. Broer, E.J. Feskens, A.J. Smit, F.A. Muskiet, J.D. Lefrandt, V.J. Bom, J.F. May, and B. Meyboom-de Jong. Effect of an increased intake of α-linolenic acid and group nutritional education on cardiovascular risk factors: the Mediterranean Alpha-linolenic Enriched Groningen Dietary Intervention (MARGARIN) study. *American Journal of Clinical Nutrition.* 2002;75(2):221-227.

Bhatnagar, D. and Durrington P.N. Omega-3 fatty acids: their role in the prevention and treatment of atherosclerosis related risk factors and complications. *International Journal of Clinical Practice.* 2003;57(4):305-514.

Bucher, H.C., P. Hengstler, C. Schindler, and G. Meier. N-3 polyunsaturated fatty acids in coronary heart disease: a meta-analysis of randomized controlled trials. *American Journal of Medicine.* 2002;112(4):298-304.

Burr, M.L., A.M. Fehily, J.F. Gilbert, S. Rogers, R.M. Holliday, P.M. Sweetnam, P.C. Elwood, and N.M. Deadman. Effects of changes in fat, fish, and fibre intakes on death and myocardial reinfarction: Diet and Reinfarction Trial (DART). *Lancet.* 1989;2(8666):757-761.

Burr, M.L., P.M. Sweetham, and A.M. Fehily. Letters to the Editor. Diet and reinfarction. *European Heart Journal.* 1994 Aug;15(8):1152-1153.

Carroll, D.N. and M.T. Roth. Evidence for the cardioprotective effects of omega-3 Fatty acids. *The Annals of Pharmacotherapy.* 2002;36(12):1950-1956.

Consumer Reports. Omega-3 Oil. Fish or Pills? Pages 30-32, July 2003

de Lorgeril, M., P. Salen, P. Defaye, P. Mabo, and F. Paillard. Dietary prevention of sudden cardiac death. *European Heart Journal.* 2002;23(4):277-285.

Din, J.N., D.E. Newby, and A.D. Flapan. Omega 3 fatty acids and cardiovascular disease—fishing for a natural treatment. *British Medical Journal.* 2004;328(7430):30-35.

Djoussé, L., S.C. Hunt, D.K. Arnett, M.A. Province, J.H. Eckfeldt, and R.C. Ellison. Dietary linolenic acid is inversely associated with plasma triacylglycerol: the National Heart, Lung, and Blood Institute Family Heart Study. *American Journal of Clinical Nutrition.* 2003;78(6):1098-1102.

Engler, M.M., M.B. Engler, M.J. Malloy, E.Y. Chiu, and M.M. Mietus-Synder. The effect of docosahexaenoic acid on lipoprotein subclasses in hyperlipidemic children: the EARLY study. Presented at the Annual Scientific Sessions of the American Heart Association, 2002, Chicago Illinois. AHA: (B) Engler, M.M., M.B. Engler, M.J. Malloy, E.Y. Chiu, M.M. Mietus-Synder, M.C. Schiotter, J.D. Marrow, R. Nader, P.M. Ridkar, and M.M. Mietus-Synder. Docosahexaenoic acid, an omega-3 fatty acid, improves endothelial function in hyperlipidemic children: Endothelial assessment of risk from lipids in youth (EARLY) study. Presented at the Annual Scientific Sessions of the American Heart Association, 2002, Chicago, Illinois. AHA.

Federal Judicial Center, Reference Manual on Scientific Evidence, Second Edition, 2000, page 93

Finnegan, Y.E., A.M. Minihane, E.C. Leigh-Firbank, S. Kew, G.W. Meijer, R. Muggli, P.C. Calder, and C.M. Williams. Plant- and marine-derived n-3 polyunsaturated fatty acids have differential effects on fasting and postprandial blood lipid concentrations and on the susceptibility of LDL to oxidative modification in moderately hyperlipidemic subjects. *American Journal of Clinical Nutrition.* 2003;77(4):783-795.

Foran, S.E., J.G. Flood, and K.B. Lewandrowski. Measurement of mercury levels in concentrated over-the-counter fish oil preparations. Is fish oil healthier than fish? *Arachives of Pathology & Laboratory Medicine.* 2003;127:1603-1605.

Forsyth, J.S., P. Willatts, C. Agostoni, J. Bissenden, P. Casaer, and G. Boehm. Long chain polyunsaturated fatty acid supplementation in infant formula and blood pressure in later childhood: follow up of a randomized controlled trial. *British Medical Journal.* 2003;326(7396):953-957.

Geleijnse, J.M., E.J. Giltay, D.E. Grobbee, A.R. Donders, and F.J. Kok. Blood pressure response to fish oil supplementation: metaregression analysis of randomized trials. *Journal of Hypertension.* 2002;20(8):1493-1499.

Ghafoorunissa, A. Vani, R. Laxmi, and B. Sesikeran. Effects of dietary alpha-linolenic acid from blended oils on biochemical indices of coronary heart disease in Indians. *Lipids.* 2002;37(11):1077-1086.

Gillum, R.F., M. Mussolino, and J.H. Madans. The relation between fish consumption, death from all causes, and incidence of coronary heart disease. The NHANES I Epidemiologic Follow-up Study. *Journal of Clinical Epidemiology.* 2000;53(3):237-244.

GISSI-Prevenzione Investigators. Dietary supplementation with n-3 polyunsaturated fatty acids and vitamin E after myocardial infarction: results of the GISSI-Prevenzione trial. *Lancet.* 1999; 354:447-455.

Grundy, S.M. N-3 fatty acids: priority for post-myocardial infarction clinical trials. *Circulation.* 2003;107(14):1834-1836.

Guallar, E., M.I. Sanz-Gallardo, P. van't Veer, P. Bode, and A. Aro, J. Gomez-Aracena, J.D. Kark, and R.A. Riemersma, J.M. Martin-Moreno, and F.J. Kok, for the Heavy Metals and Myocardial Infarction Study Group. Mercury, fish oils, and the risk of myocardial infarction. *The New England Journal of Medicine.* 2002;347(22):1747-1754.

Hallgren, C.G., G. Hallmans, J.H. Jansson, S.L. Marklund, F. Huhtasaari, A. Schütz, U. Strömberg, B. Vessby, and S. Skerfving. Markers of high fish intake are associated with decreased risk of a first myocardial infarction. *British Journal of Nutrition.* 2001;86(3):397-404.

Holub, B.J. Clinical nutrition: 4. Omega-3 fatty acids in cardiovascular care. *Canadian Medical Association Journal.* 2002;166(5):608-615.

Hu, F.B., L. Bronner, W.C. Willett, M.J. Stampfer, K.M. Rexrode, C.M. Albert, D. Hunter, and J.E. Manson. Fish and ω-3 fatty acid intake and risk of coronary heart disease in women. *Journal of the American Medical Association.* 2002;287(14):1815-1821.

Hu, F.B. and W.C. Willett. Optimal diets for prevention of coronary heart disease. *Journal of the American Medical Association.* 2002;288(20):2569-2578.

Hu, F.B., E. Cho, K.M. Rexrode, C.M. Albert, and J.E. Manson. Fish and long-chain ω-3 fatty acid intake and risk of coronary heart disease and total mortality in diabetic women. *Circulation.* 2003;107(14):1852-1857.

Institute of Medicine of the National Academies, Dietary Reference Intakes for Energy, Carbohydrate, Fiber, Fat, Fatty Acids, Cholesterol, Protein and Amino Acids. Chapter 8, "Dietary Fats: Total Fat and Fatty Acids," and Chapter 11, "Macronutrients and Healthful Diets," (National Academy Press 2002).

Izzat, L.M. and P. Avery. What is the current role of omega-3 polyunsaturated fatty acids in post-myocardial infarction management? *British Journal of Cardiology.* 2002;9:600-609.

Kris-Etherton, P.M., W.S. Harris, and L.J. Appel; American Heart Association. Nutrition Committee. Fish consumption, fish oil, omega-3 fatty acids, and cardiovascular disease. *Circulation.* 2002;106(21):2747-2757.

Kris-Etherton, P.M., W.S. Harris, and L.J. Appel; Nutrition Committee. Fish consumption, fish oil, omega-3 fatty acids, and cardiovascular disease. *Arteriosclerosis, Thrombosis, and Vascular Biology.* 2003;23(2):151-152.

Krokan, H.E., K.S. Bjerve, and E. Mørk. The enteral bioavailability of eicosapentaenoic acid and docosahexaenoic acid is good from ethyl esters as from glyceryl esters in spite of lower hydrolytic rates by pancreatic lipase in vitro. *Biochimica et Biophysica Acta.* 1993;1168(1):59-67.

Laidlaw, M. and B.J. Holub. Effects of supplementation with fish oil-derived n-3 fatty acids and γ-linolenic acid on circulating plasma lipids and fatty acid profiles in women. *American Journal of Clinical Nutrition.* 2003;77(1):37-42.

Lanzmann-Petithory, D, S. Pueyo, and S. Renaud. Primary prevention of cardiovascular diseases by alpha-linolenic acid. *American Journal of Clinical Nutrition.* 2002;76(6):1456.

Leaf, A., J.X. Kang, Y.F. Xiao, and G.E. Billman. Clinical prevention of sudden cardiac death by n-3 polyunsaturated fatty acids and mechanism of prevention of arrhythmias by n-3 fish oils. *Circulation.* 2003;107(21):2646-2652.

Lemaitre, R.N., I.B. King, D. Mozaffarian, L.H. Kuller, R.P. Tracy, and D.S. Siscovick. n-3 Polyunsaturated fatty acids, fatal ischemic heart disease, and nonfatal myocardial infarction in older adults: the Cardiovascular

Health Study. *American Journal of Clinical Nutrition.* 2003; 77(2):319-325.

Leng, G.C., A.J. Lee, F.G. Fowkes, R.G. Jepson, G.D. Lowe, E.R. Skinner, and B.F. Mowat. Randomized controlled trial of gamma-linolenic acid and eicosapentaenoic acid in peripheral arterial disease. *Clinical Nutrition.* 1998;17(6):265-271.

Marchioli, R., F. Barzi, E. Bomba, C. Chieffo, D. Di Gregorio, R. Di Mascio, M.G. Franzosi, E. Geraci, G. Levantesi, A.P. Maggioni, L. Mantini, R.M. Marfisi, G. Mastrogiuseppe, N. Mininni, G.L. Nicolosi, M. Santini, C. Schweiger, L. Tavazzi, G. Tognoni, C. Tucci, and F. Valagussa; GISSI-Prevenzione Investigators. Early protection against sudden death by n-3 polyunsaturated fatty acids after myocardial infarction: time-course analysis of the results of the Gruppo Italiano per lo Studio della Sopravvivenza nell'Infarto Miocardico (GISSI)-Prevenzione. *Circulation.* 2002;105(16):1897-1903.

Maresta, A., M. Balduccelli, E. Varani, M. Marzilli, C. Galli, F. Heiman, M. Lavezzari, E. Stragliotto, and R. De Caterina; ESPRIT Investigators. Prevention of postcoronary angioplasty restenosis by omega-3 fatty acids: main results of the Esapent for Prevention of Restenosis ITalian Study (ESPRIT). *American Heart Journal.* 2002;143(6):E5.

Morris D.H. Methodologic challenges in designing clinical studies to measure differences in the bioequivalence of n-3 fatty acids. *Molecular and Cellular Biochemistry.* 2003;246(1-2):83-90.

Mozaffarian, D., R.N. Lemaitre, L.H. Kuller, G.L. Burke, R.P. Tracy, and D.S. Siscovick; Cardiovascular Health Study. Cardiac benefits of fish consumption may depend on the type of fish meal consumed: the Cardiovascular Health Study. *Circulation.* 2003;107(10):1372-1377.

Nilsen, D.W., G. Albrektsen, K. Landmark, S. Moen, T. Aarsland, and L. Woie. Effects of a high-dose concentrate of n-3 fatty acids or corn oil introduced early after an acute myocardial infarction on serum triacylglycerol and HDL cholesterol. *American Journal of Clinical Nutrition.* 2001;74(1):50-56.

Nordøy, A. Statins and omega-3 fatty acids in the treatment of dyslipidemia and coronary heart disease. *Minerva Medica.* 2002;93(5):357-363.

ORC Macro. Consumer reactions to the draft advisory on methyl mercury in fish. Focus Group Research. Summary of key findings. U.S. Food and Drug Administration. March 2003.

Osler, M., A.H. Andreasen, and S. Hoidrup. No inverse association between fish consumption and risk of death from all-causes, and incidence of coronary heart disease in middle-aged, Danish adults. *Journal of Clinical Epidemiology.* 2003;56(3):274-279.

Rissanen, T., S. Voutilainen, K. Nyyssönen, T.A. Lakka, and J.T. Salonen. Fish oil-derived fatty acids, docosahexaenoic acid and docosapentaenoic acid, and the risk of acute coronary events: the Kuopio Ischaemic Heart Disease Risk Factor Study. *Circulation.* 2000;102(22):2677-2679.

Sacks, F.M., P.H. Stone, C.M. Gibson, D.I. Silverman, B. Rosner, and R.C. Pasternak. Controlled trial of fish oil for regression of human coronary atherosclerosis. HARP Research Group. *Journal of the American College of Cardiology.* 1995;25(7):1492-1498.

Sacks, F.M. and M. Katan. Randomized clinical trials on the effects of dietary fat and carbohydrate on plasma lipoproteins and cardiovascular disease. *American Journal of Medicine.* 2002;113 Suppl 9B:13S-24S.

Salonen, J.T., K. Seppänen, K. Nyyssönen, H. Korpela, J. Kauhanen, M. Kantola, J. Tuomilehto, H. Esterbauer, F. Tatzber, and R. Salonen. Intake of mercury from fish, lipid peroxidation, and the risk of myocardial infarction and coronary, cardiovascular, and any death in Eastern Finnish men. *Circulation.* 1995;91:645-655.

Singh, R.B., M.A. Niaz, J.P. Sharma, R. Kumar, V. Rastogi, and M. Moshiri. Randomized, double-blind, placebo-controlled trial of fish oil and mustard oil in patients with suspected acute myocardial infarction: the Indian Experiment of Infarct Survival—4. *Cardiovascular Drugs and Therapy.* 1997;11(3):485-491.

Singh, R.B., G. Dubnov, M.A. Niaz, S. Ghosh, R. Singh, S.S. Rastogi, O. Manor, D. Pella, and E.M. Berry. Effect of an Indo-Mediterranean diet on progression of coronary artery disease in high risk patients (Indo-Mediterranean Diet Heart Study): a randomized single-blind trial. *Lancet.* 2002;360(9344):1455-1461.

Siscovick, D.S., R.N. Lemaitre, and D. Mozaffarian. The fish story: a diet-heart hypothesis with clinical implications: n-3 polyunsaturated fatty acids, myocardial vulnerability, and sudden death. *Circulation.* 2003;107(21):2632-2634.

Skerrett, P.J. and C.H. Hennekens. Consumption of fish and fish oils and decreased risk of stroke. *Preventive Cardiology.* 2003;6(1):38-41.

Spilker, B. Guide to Clinical Studies. Raven Press, New York, New York, 1991. Pages 15, 62, 793.

Thies, F., J.M. Garry, P. Yaqoob, K. Rerkasem, J. Williams, C.P. Shearman, P.J. Gallagher, P.C. Calder, and R.F. Grimble. Association of n-3 polyunsaturated fatty acids with stability of atherosclerotic plaques: a randomized controlled trial. *Lancet.* 2003;361(9356):477-485.

Torres, I.C., L. Mira, C.P. Ornelas, and A. Melim. Study of the effects of dietary fish intake on serum lipids and lipoproteins in two populations with different dietary habits. *British Journal of Nutrition.* 2000;83(4):371-379.

United States Department of Agriculture and United States Department of Health and Human Services. Nutrition and Your Health: Dietary Guidelines for Americans. Fifth Edition, 2000. Home and Garden Bulletin No. 232, 2000.

United States Department of Health and Human Services. Detection, Evaluation, and Treatment of High Blood Cholesterol in Adults (Adult Treatment Panel III). Executive Summary. NIH Publication No. 01-3670. 2001.

von Schacky, C., P. Angerer, W. Kothny, K. Theisen, and H. Mudra. The effect of dietary ω-3 fatty acids on coronary atherosclerosis. A randomized, double-blind, placebo-controlled trial. *Annals of Internal Medicine.* 1999;130(7):554-562.

Woodman, R.J., T.A. Mori, V. Burke, I.B. Puddey, G.F. Watts, and L.J. Beilin. Effects of purified eicosapentaenoic and docosahexaenoic acids on glycemic control, blood pressure, and serum lipids in type 2 diabetic patients with treated hypertension. *American Journal of Clinical Nutrition.* 2002;76(5):1007-1015.

Yoshizawa, K., E.B. Rimm, J.S. Morris, V.L. Spate, C.C. Hsieh, D. Spiegelman, M.J. Stampfer, and W.C. Willett. Mercury and the risk of coronary heart disease in men. *The New England Journal of Medicine.* 2002;347(22):1755-1760.

ENDNOTES

[1]   "Interim Procedures for Qualified Health Claims in the Labeling of Conventional Human Food and Human Dietary Supplements" that published on July 10, 2003. http://www.cfsan.fda.gov/~dms/nuttf-e.html.

[2]   A letter from Christine J. Lewis, Ph.D., FDA to Jonathan W. Emord, Esq., Emord & Associates, P.C., "Letter Regarding Dietary Supplement Health Claim for Omega-3 Fatty Acids and Coronary Heart Disease" (Docket No. 91N-0103), October 31, 2000. http://www.cfsan.fda.gov/~dms/ds-ltr11.html.

[3]   A letter from Christine J. Lewis, Ph.D., FDA to Jonathan W. Emord, Esq., Emord & Associates, P.C., "Letter Clarifying Conditions for a

Dietary Supplement Health Claim for Omega-3 Fatty Acids and Coronary Heart Disease" (Docket No. 91N-0103), February 16, 2001. http://www.cfsan.fda.gov/~dms/ds-ltr20.html.

[4]   A letter from Christine J. Taylor, Ph.D., FDA to Jonathan W. Emord, Esq., Emord & Associates, P.C., "Letter Responding to a Request to Reconsider the Qualified Claim for Dietary Supplement Health Claim for Omega-3 Fatty Acids and Coronary Heart Disease" (Docket No. 91N-0103), February 8, 2002. http://www.cfsan.fda.gov/~dms/ds-ltr28.html.

[5]   See footnote 2.

[6]   See footnote 3.

[7]   See footnote 4.

[8]   This guidance published on July 10, 2003. http://www.cfsan.fda.gov/~dms/nuttf-b.html.

[9]   A meta-analysis is the process of systematically combining and evaluating the results of clinical trials that have been completed or terminated (i.e., primary reports) (Spilker, 1991). FDA uses meta-analyses to identify relevant primary reports, which the Agency then evaluates individually.

[10] Review articles summarize the findings of primary reports. FDA uses review articles to identify primary reports that are relevant for review. FDA also uses review articles to identify information that is useful to understand the scientific issues about the substance-disease relationship (i.e., used as background information).

[11] The physiology of animals is different than that of humans, thus animals often respond differently to dietary interventions compared to humans.

[12] *In vitro* studies are conducted in an artificial environment and cannot account for a multitude of normal physiological processes such as digestion, absorption, distribution, and metabolism that affect how humans respond to the consumption of foods and dietary substances. Therefore, *in vitro* studies generally are not able to provide scientific evidence about the relationship between a substance and disease risk.

[13] Angerer et al., 2002; Finnegan et al., 2003; Ghafoorunissa et al., 2002; Laidlaw and Holub 2003; Thies et al., 2003; Woodman et al., 2002.

[14] Albert et al., 2002; Gillum et al., 2000; Hu et al., 2003; Lamaitre et al., 2003; Mozaffarian et al., 2003; Osler et al., 2003 ; Torres et al. 2000.

[15] Baylin et al., 2003; Bemelmans et al., 2002; Djoussé et al., 2003; Forsyth et al., 2003; Singh et al., 2002.

[16]   Ascherio 2002; Bhatnagar and Durrington, 2003; Carroll and Roth, 2002; de Lorgeril and Salen, 2002; Grundy 2003; Harris et al., 2003; Holub 2002; Hu and Willet, 2002; Izzat and Avery, 2002; Leaf et al., 2003; Nordøy 2002; Sacks and Katan, 2002; Skerrett and Hennekens, 2003.

[17]   Bucher et al., 2002; Geleijnse et al., 2002.

[18]   Kris-Etherton et al., 2002.

[19]   Kris-Etherton et al., 2003; Lanzmann-Petithory et al., 2002; Morris, 2003; Siscovick et al., 2003.

[20]   Institute of Medicine, 2002.

[21]   Guallar et al., 2002; Yoshizawa et al., 2002.

[22]   Engler et al., 2002.

[23]   Burr et al., 1994 (also Burr et al., 1989); GISSI-Prevenzione Investigators,1999; Marchioli et al., 2002; Maresta et al., 2002; Singh et al., 1997.

[24]   Leng et al., 1998.

[25]   Nilsen et al. 2001.

[26]   Albert et al. 1998; Hallgren et al., 2001; Hu et al., 2002; Rissanen et al., 2000.

[27]   U.S. Department of Agriculture, Agricultural Research Service. 2004. USDA National Nutrient Database for Standard Reference, Release 17 (http://www.nal.usda.gov/fnic/foodcomp/Data/SR17/sr17.html).

[28]   Summary of all GRAS notices. http://www.cfsan.fda.gov/~rdb/opa-gras.html.

[29]   Institute of Medicine of the National Academies. Dietary Reference Intakes. Energy, Carbohydrate, Fiber, Fat, Fatty Acids, Cholesterol, Protein, and Amino Acids. Part 2. Pages E-13, E-14. http://www.nap.edu/books/0309085373/html/.

[30]   Conventional foods enriched with EPA and DHA containing food ingredients are not included in the estimates.

[31]   See footnote 2.

[32]   National Heart, Blood and Lung Institute (NHLBI), Heart and Blood Vessel Diseases (http://www.nhlbi.nih.gov/health/dci/Diseases/Atherosclerosis/Atherosclerosis_WhatIs.html) and National Cholesterol Education Program, Page 3 (U.S. Department of Health and Human Services, 2001, http://www.nhlbi.nih.gov/guidelines/cholesterol/atp_iii.htm).

[33]   See footnote 32.

[34]   See footnote 2.

[35] Albert et al., 1998; Burr et al., 1994 (also Burr et al., 1989); GISSI-Prevenzione Investigators,1999; Singh et al., 1997.

[36] Angerer et al., 2002; Finnegan et al., 2003; Ghafoorunissa et al., 2002; Laidlaw and Holub 2003; Thies et al., 2003; Woodman et al., 2002.

[37] Marchioli et al., 2002; Maresta et al., 2002.

[38] Leng et al., 1998.

[39] Nilsen et al. 2001.

[40] Neither the patient/subject nor the investigator is aware of which treatment the patient/subject is receiving (Spilker, 1991).

[41] FDA considers the subjects in this study to be representative of the general population because they did not have CHD and the physiological responses to omega-3 fatty acids is the same in hyperlipidemics and normolipidemics (reviewed in the 2000 letter).

[42] FDA considered this study relevant to its review because the bioavailability and distribution of EPA ethyl ester and DHA ethyl esters are equivalent to the natural forms of EPA and DHA from fish oil (Krokan, et al., 1993).

[43] Diabetes is a risk factor for CHD (What Makes a Heart Attach More Likely? National Institutes of Health, National Heart, Lung, and Blood   Institute (http://www.nhlbi.nih.gov/health/dci/Diseases/HeartAttack/heartattac k_risk.html). FDA considers this study on diabetics relevant to its review for establishing the substance-disease relationship because: (1) the diabetic study population did not have CHD and; (2) omega-3 fatty acids affect blood pressure in diabetics and healthy individuals similarly (Evidence Report/Technology Assessment: Number 94, Effects of Omega-3 Fatty Acids on Cardiovascular Disease, Agency for Healthcare Research and Quality, March 2004, page 63-64, http://www.ahrq.gov/clinic/evrptfiles.htm#o3cardio).

[44] Gillum et al., 2000; Hu et al., 2003; Mozaffarian et al., 2003; Osler et al., 2003.

[45] Hu et al., 2002; Rissanen et al., 2000.

[46] Albert et al., 2002; Lamaitre et al., 2003.

[47] Hallgren et al., 2001.

[48] Torres et al., 2000.

[49] Gillum et al., 2000; Osler et al., 2003.

[50] Not all fish contain significant amounts of EPA and DHA omega-3 fatty acids (see footnote 27).

[51] Albert et al., 1998, 2002 ; Hallgren et al., 2001; Hu et al., 2002 ; Hu et al., 2003; Lamaitre et al.,2003; Mozaffarian et al., 2003 ; Rissanen et al., 2000; Torres et al., 2000.

[52] Quintiles are values that divide a sample of data into five groups containing (as far as possible) equal numbers of observations.

[53] DPA, docosapentaenoic acid, is formed from EPA and is converted to DHA.

[54] Ischemic heart disease is a form of coronary heart disease (CHD).

[55] A method of dietary assessment in which subjects are asked to recall how frequently certain foods were consumed during a specified period of time.

[56] Dietary Reference Intakes for Energy, Carbohydrate, Fiber, Fat, Fatty Acids, Cholesterol, Protein, and Amino Acids, Part 2, Chapter 11, Page 11-40 (Institutes of the Medicine of the National Academies, 2002).

[57] Guidance for Industry: Significant Scientific Agreement in the Review of Health Claims for Conventional Foods and Dietary Supplements, December 22, 1999 (http://www.cfsan.fda.gov/~dms/ ssaguide.html).

[58] See footnote 2.

[59] Telephone communication with Martin J. Hahn on August 24, 2004.

[60] See footnote 2.

[61] See footnote 3.

[62] See footnote 4.

[63] See footnote 59.

[64] See footnote 59.

[65] See footnote 59.

[66] See footnote 4.

[67] See footnote 2.

[68] See footnote 28.

[69] U.S. Department of Health and Human Services and U.S. Environmental Protection Agency, "What You Need to Know About Mercury in Fish and Shellfish, 2004 EPA and FDA Advice For: Women Who Might Become Pregnant, Women Who are Pregnant, Nursing Mothers, Young Children." March 2004. http://www. cfsan.fda.gov/~dms/admehg3.html.

[70] See, e.g., *UAW v. Chao*, 361 F.3d 249 (3rd Cir. 2004), (court deferred to OSHA's decision to pursue various non-regulatory measures, such as non-mandatory guidelines and educational programs, rather than to promulgate a rule limiting worker exposure to metalworking fluids,

which were acknowledged by the court to have debilitating health effects); *CFA v. CPSC*, 990 F.2d 1298 (DC Cir. 1993), (court deferred to CPSC's decision to negotiate a comprehensive consent decree with vehicle manufacturers and dealer monitoring agreements, rather than to promulgate a rule banning the sale of all-terrain vehicles for use by children under the age of sixteen. The court stated: "We accord due respect, moreover, to an agency's selection of means for pursuing policy goals. Such choices implicate the allocation of scarce administrative resources; they involve forecasts about the consequences of proposed regulatory actions and other matters the agency ordinarily is best equipped to judge.").

[71] For instance, with regard to the mercury in fish advisory, the agency is targeting mailings about the advisory to appropriate health professionals, e.g., obstetrician - gynecologists. The agency is also targeting the appropriate media, e.g., women's magazines, as well as professional health organizations that deal with pregnant women, women who might become pregnant, nursing mothers and young children.

Chapter 3

EFFECTS OF OMEGA-3 FATTY ACIDS ON LIPIDS AND GLYCEMIC CONTROL IN TYPE II DIABETES AND THE METABOLIC SYNDROME AND ON INFLAMMATORY BOWEL DISEASE, RHEUMATOID ARTHRITIS, RENAL DISEASE, SYSTEMIC LUPUS ERYTHEMATOSUS, AND OSTEOPOROSIS

ABSTRACT

Under its Evidence-based Practice Program, the Agency for Healthcare Research and Quality (AHRQ) is developing scientific information for other agencies and organizations on which to base clinical guidelines, performance measures, and other quality improvement tools. Contractor institutions review all relevant scientific literature on assigned clinical care topics and produce evidence reports and technology assessments, conduct research on methodologies and the effectiveness of their implementation, and participate in technical assistance activities.

INTRODUCTION

This report was requested and funded by the Office of Dietary Supplements, National Institutes of Health. It is one of several reports focusing on the role of omega-3 fatty acids in the prevention or treatment of various diseases. Three Evidence-based Practice Centers (EPCs) produced this series of reports: the Southern California EPC, based at RAND, the Tufts-New England Medical Center EPC, and the University of Ottawa EPC. This particular report focuses on the effects of omega-3 fatty acids on immune-mediated diseases, bone metabolism, and gastrointestinal/renal diseases.

Over the past 40 years, an increasing number of physiological functions have been attributed to omega-3 fatty acids, including movement of calcium and other substances into and out of cells, relaxation and contraction of muscles, inhibition and promotion of clotting, regulation of secretion of substances that include digestive enzymes and hormones, control of fertility, cell division, and growth. [1] In addition, omega-3 fatty acids may play an important role in brain development and function. Some evidence has suggested that omega-3 fatty acids in the diet may protect against heart attack and stroke, as well as certain inflammatory diseases like arthritis, lupus, and asthma. [1] The major dietary sources of omega-3 fatty acids in the U.S. population are fish, fish oil, vegetable oils (principally canola and soybean), walnuts, wheat germ, and some dietary supplements.

METHODS

Key Questions

We consulted with three technical expert panels (TEPs) on this project. The respective panels focused on the following conditions:

- Rheumatoid arthritis, systemic lupus erythematosis (SLE), and bone density/osteoporosis.
- Renal disease and diabetes.
- Gastrointestinal diseases.

The TEPs advised us on refining the preliminary questions posed to us by AHRQ, determining the proper inclusion/exclusion criteria for the study and the populations of interest, establishing the proper outcomes measures, and conducting the appropriate analyses.

Based on the original questions that we received from AHRQ and input from our TEPs, we addressed the following questions in this study:

Diabetes

- What is the evidence in adults or children with a) type II diabetes, or b) insulin resistance/the metabolic syndrome for an effect of omega-3 fatty acids on:
  - Total cholesterol.
  - HDL cholesterol.
  - LDL cholesterol.
  - Triglycerides.
- What is the evidence in adults and children for an effect of omega-3 fatty acids on insulin sensitivity in a) type II diabetes, or b) the metabolic syndrome?

Inflammatory Bowel Disease

- What is the evidence for the efficacy of omega-3 fatty acids in treatment of Crohn's disease and ulcerative colitis?
- What is the evidence in adults or children with inflammatory bowel disease that omega-3 fatty acids can replace steroids or other immunosuppressive drugs?
- What is the evidence that the benefits of omega-3 fatty acids are influenced by the concomitant administration of various immunosuppressive agents in the treatment of inflammatory bowel disease?

Rheumatoid Arthritis

- What is the evidence in adults or children with rheumatoid arthritis that omega-3 fatty acids affect:
  - Pain.
  - Number of swollen joints.

- – Disease activity.
- – Patients' global assessment.
- – Joint damage.
- What is the evidence in adults or children with rheumatoid arthritis that omega-3 fatty acids can replace other more potent anti-inflammatory or immunosuppressive drugs such as steroids and nonsteroidal anti-inflammatory drugs?
- What is the evidence that the benefits of omega-3 fatty acids are influenced by the concomitant administration of various immunosuppressive agents in the treatment of rheumatoid arthritis?

Renal Disease

- What is the evidence for the efficacy of omega-3 fatty acids in treatment of renal inflammation and glomerulosclerosis?
- What is the evidence in adults or children with immune-mediated renal disease that omega-3 fatty acids can replace steroids or other immunosuppressive drugs?
- What is the evidence that the benefits of omega-3 fatty acids are influenced by the concomitant administration of various immunosuppressive agents in the treatment of immune-mediated renal disease?

Systemic Lupus Erythematosus

- What is the evidence in adults or children with SLE that omega-3 fatty acids affect disease activity, damage, or patient perceptions of outcomes in SLE?
- What is the evidence in adults or children with SLE that omega-3 fatty acids can replace steroids or other immunosuppressive drugs?
- What is the evidence that the benefits of omega-3 fatty acids in the treatment of SLE are influenced by the concomitant administration of various immunosuppressive agents?

Bone Density/Osteoporosis

–   What is the evidence that omega-3 fatty acids help maintain bone mineral status?

For each of the study questions, we also assessed:

–   The effect of omega-3 fatty acids on subpopulations.
–   The effects of covariates, dose, source, and exposure duration on the outcomes of interest.
–   The sustainment of effect.

In addition to answering these questions, we evaluated the data on adverse events, including clinical bleeding, gastrointestinal complaints or nausea, diarrhea, headache, dermatological problems, and withdrawal from study due to an adverse event.

Search Strategy

We searched the following online databases to identify literature:

–   MEDLINE® (1966-July 2003).
–   PreMEDLINE® (July 8, 2003).
–   EMBASE (1980-Week 27, 2003).
–   Cochrane Central Register of Controlled Trials (2nd Quarter, 2003).
–   CAB Health® (1973-June 2003).
–   Dissertation Abstracts (1861-December 2002).

We developed a core search strategy and applied it to each relevant disease category:

–   Rheumatoid arthritis.
–   Bone density.
–   SLE.
–   Renal disease.
–   Diabetes.
–   Gastrointestinal diseases.

We also reviewed the reference lists of all applicable articles and contacted our technical expert panel as well as industry experts to identify unpublished data.

Selection Criteria

Two reviewers independently reviewed each article considered for inclusion in the study. Any disagreements between the reviewers were resolved through consensus. We included any articles pertaining to the effects of omega-3 fatty acids on diabetes mellitus, inflammatory bowel disease (ulcerative colitis and Crohn's disease), rheumatoid arthritis, SLE, renal disease, osteoporosis, or bone mineral status. We included only articles that presented research on human subjects and those that reported the results of randomized clinical trials or controlled clinical trials; we accepted observational studies only for bone mineral status. Language was not a barrier to inclusion.

Data Extraction and Analysis

For each article included in the study, two reviewers independently extracted data about:

- The trial design.
- The outcomes of interest.
- The quality of the trial.
- The number and characteristics of the patients.
- Details on the intervention, such as the dose, frequency, and duration.
- The types of outcome measures.
- Adverse events.
- The elapsed time between the intervention and outcome measurements.

Any disagreements between the reviewers were resolved through consensus. For each article, we then evaluated the quality of the design and execution of trials using a system developed by Jadad; determined a combined applicability grade based on applicability to the U.S. population and health state; performed a meta-analysis of those studies that sufficiently assessed interventions, populations, and outcomes to justify pooling; and performed a qualitative analysis of the remaining studies.

RESULTS

We screened 4,212 article titles. From these article titles, we reviewed the 1,097 full-text articles relevant to our topics. Of these full-text articles, 115 met our selection criteria and underwent detailed review; among these, 83 articles met our inclusion criteria (34 for diabetes/metabolic syndrome, 13 for inflammatory bowel disease, 21 for rheumatoid arthritis, 9 for renal disease, 3 for SLE, and 4 for bone density and fractures). All of these 83 articles were randomized controlled trials, except for one observational study of bone density. We had a sufficient number of articles to perform quantitative meta-analyses for rheumatoid arthritis, inflammatory bowel disease, and diabetes. Due to the limited number of articles we identified for renal failure, SLE, and bone mineral metabolism, we performed qualitative analyses for these conditions.

Overall, our analyses yielded variable results both within and among disease categories. Our findings are summarized for each condition studied.

Diabetes/Metabolic Syndrome

Among 18 studies of type II diabetes or the metabolic syndrome, omega-3 fatty acids had a favorable effect on triglyceride levels relative to placebo (pooled random effects estimate: -31.61; 95% CI, -49.58, -13.64) but had no effect on total cholesterol, HDL cholesterol, LDL cholesterol, fasting blood sugar, or glycosylated hemoglobin, by meta-analysis. Omega-3 fatty acids had no effect on plasma insulin or insulin resistance in type II diabetics or patients with the metabolic syndrome, by qualitative analysis of four studies.

Inflammatory Bowel Disease

Among 13 studies reporting outcomes in patients with inflammatory bowel disease, variable effects of omega-3 fatty acids on clinical score, sigmoidoscopic score, histologic score, induced remission, and relapse were reported. In ulcerative colitis, omega-3 fatty acids had no effect on the relative risk of relapse in a meta-analysis of three studies. There was a statistically non-significant reduction in requirement for corticosteroids for omega-3 fatty acids relative to placebo in two studies. No studies evaluated the effect of omega-3 fatty acids on requirement for other immunosuppressive agents.

Rheumatoid Arthritis

Among nine studies reporting outcomes in patients with rheumatoid arthritis, omega-3 fatty acids had no effect on patient report of pain, swollen joint count, Erythrocyte Sedimentation Rate (ESR), and patient's global assessment by meta-analysis. A previously performed meta-analysis[2] reached the same conclusions for swollen joint count, ESR, and patient's global assessment. That meta-analysis found a statistically significant improvement in tender joint count compared to placebo (rate difference = -2.9, 95% CI, -3.8, -2.1). The one study that assessed the effect on joint damage found no effect. In a qualitative analysis of seven studies that assessed the effect of omega-3 fatty acids on anti-inflammatory drug or corticosteriod requirement, six demonstrated reduced requirement for these drugs. No studies assessed the effect on requirements for disease modifying anti-rheumatic drugs. None of the studies used a composite score that incorporates both subjective and objective measures of disease activity, such as the American College of Rheumatology response criteria.

Renal Disease

In a qualitative analysis of nine studies that assessed the effect of omega-3 fatty acids in renal disease, there were varying effects on serum creatinine and creatinine clearance and no effect on progression to end stage renal disease. In a single study that assessed the effect on hemodialysis graft patency, graft patency was significantly better with fish oil than with placebo. No studies assessed the effects of omega-3 fatty acids on requirements for corticosteroids.

Systemic Lupus Erythematosis

Among three studies that assessed the effects of omega-3 fatty acids in SLE, variable effects on clinical activity were reported. No studies were identified that assessed effect on damage or patient perception of disease. Omega-3 fatty acids had no effect on corticosteroid requirements in one study. No studies were identified that assessed the effects of omega-3 fatty acids on requirements for other immunosuppressive drugs for SLE. None of the studies used a measure of disease activity that incorporates both subjective and objective measures of disease activity.

Bone Mineral Density/Fracture

Among five studies described in four reports the effect of omega-3 fatty acids on bone mineral density was variable. No studies that assessed the effect of omega-3 fatty acids on fracture were identified.

The quantity and strength of evidence for effects of omega-3 fatty acids on outcomes in the conditions assessed varies greatly. The findings of many studies among type II diabetics provide strong evidence that omega-3 fatty acids reduce serum triglycerides but have no effect on total cholesterol, HDL cholesterol, and LDL cholesterol. For rheumatoid arthritis, the available evidence suggests that omega-3 fatty acids reduce tender joint counts and may reduce requirements for corticosteroids, but does not support an effect of omega-3 fatty acids on other clinical outcomes. There are insufficient data available to draw conclusions about the effects of omega-3 fatty acids on inflammatory bowel disease, renal disease, SLE, bone density, or fractures or the effects of omega-3 fatty acids on insulin resistance among type II diabetics.

DISCUSSION

We offer the following observations and recommendations regarding future research on the effects of omega-3 fatty acids on lipids and glycemic control in type II diabetes and the metabolic syndrome and on inflammatory bowel disease, rheumatoid arthritis, renal disease, SLE, and osteoporosis:

- Additional research on the effects of omega-3 fatty acids needs to be performed on inflammatory bowel disease, renal disease, SLE, bone density, or fractures or the effects of omega-3 fatty acids on insulin resistance among type II diabetics before recommendations regarding the use of omega-3 fatty acids for these conditions can be made.
- Studies of inflammatory bowel disease that include patients with both Crohn's disease and ulcerative colitis should report data separately for these groups.
- Studies that assess the effects of omega-3 fatty acids should use standard validated instruments to assess clinical outcomes.
- Trials that assess the effects of omega-3 fatty acids should be designed to evaluate the effect of source, dose, treatment duration, and the sustainment of effect after discontinuation of omega-3 fatty acid consumption.
- Studies of omega-3 fatty acids should explicitly define both the quantity of the omega-3 fatty acid source and of the specific omega-3 fatty acids present in a study dose of that source.
- Trials of omega-3 fatty acids should include a baseline assessment of dietary omega-3 and omega-6 fatty acid intake.
- In controlled trials that assess the effects of omega-3 fatty acids, analysis should include and report explicit testing of the effects of the omega-3 fatty acid relative to the control substance.
- In studies that use a crossover design, outcome data for all study arms should be reported at the end of each treatment period.

AVAILABILITY OF FULL REPORT

The full evidence report from which this summary was taken was prepared for the Agency for Healthcare Research and Quality (AHRQ) by the Southern California/RAND Evidence-based Practice Center, Los Angeles, CA, under Contract No. 290-02-0003. Printed copies may be obtained free of charge from the AHRQ Publications Clearinghouse by calling 800-358-9295. Requesters should ask for Evidence Report/Technology Assessment No. 89, *Effects of Omega-3 Fatty Acids on Lipids and Glycemic Control in Type II Diabetes and the Metabolic Syndrome and on Inflammatory Bowel Disease, Rheumatoid Arthritis, Renal Disease, Systemic Lupus Erythematosus, and Osteoporosis.*

REFERENCES

[1] Innis S. Essential dietary lipids. In: Ziegler EE, Filer, LJ Jr, editors. *Present Knowledge in Nutrition.* Washington, DC: International Life Sciences Institute; 1996.

[2] Fortin P, Lew R, Liang M, et al. Validation of a meta-analysis: The effects of fish oil in rheumatoid arthritis. *J Clin Epidemiol* 1995;48(11):1379-90.

Chapter 4

SUBSTANCES AFFIRMED AS GENERALLY RECOGNIZED AS SAFE: MENHADEN OIL

ABSTRACT

The Food and Drug Administration (FDA) is issuing a tentative final rule to amend its regulations by reallocating the uses of menhaden oil in food that currently are established in Sec. 184.1472 (21 CFR 184.1472). FDA has tentatively concluded that these uses of menhaden oil are generally recognized as safe (GRAS), but only when the menhaden oil is not used in combination with other added oils that are significant sources of eicosapentaenoic acid (EPA) and docosahexaenoic acid (DHA). Because FDA's proposed rule of February 26, 2002, did not include a condition of use for other added oils, FDA is issuing this tentative final rule to give interested persons an opportunity to comment on this use limitation.

I. BACKGROUND

Menhaden oil is a refined marine oil that is derived from menhaden fish (Brevoortia species). Menhaden oil differs from edible vegetable oils and animal fats in its high proportion of polyunsaturated fatty acids, including omega-3 fatty acids. EPA and DHA are the major source of omega-3 fatty acids from fish oil and together comprise approximately 20 percent by weight of menhaden oil. In response to a petition (GRASP 6G0316) from the National Fish Meal and Oil Association, FDA issued a final rule on June 5, 1997 (62 FR 30751) (the June 1997 final rule), affirming menhaden oil as

GRAS for use as a direct human food ingredient with limitations on the maximum use levels of menhaden oil in specific food categories. FDA concluded that these limitations are necessary to ensure that daily intakes of EPA and DHA from menhaden oil do not exceed 3.0 grams per person per day (g/p/d). As discussed in the following paragraphs, the maximum limit of 3.0 g/p/ d on the total daily intake of EPA and DHA is a safeguard against the possible effects of these fatty acids on increased bleeding time (the time taken for bleeding from a standardized skin wound to cease), glycemic control in non-insulin-dependent diabetics, and increased levels of low-density lipoprotein (LDL) cholesterol. The concerns over possible adverse effects of fish oil consumption on bleeding time, glycemic control, and LDL cholesterol were discussed in the June 1997 final rule.

As part of FDA's evaluation of GRASP 6G0316, FDA examined the scientific literature for evidence that consumption of fish oils may contribute to excessive bleeding. In the June 1997 final rule, FDA concluded based on this examination of the scientific literature, including more than 50 reports on fish oils with data on bleeding time, that when consumption of fish oils is limited to 3.0 g/p/d or less of EPA and DHA, there is no significant risk for increased bleeding time beyond the normal range (62 FR 30751 at 30752 to 30753). FDA also concluded that amounts of fish oils providing more than 3.0 g/p/d of EPA and DHA have generally been found to produce increases in bleeding time that are statistically significant, but that there are insufficient data to evaluate the clinical significance of this finding. Therefore, because of the lack of data on clinical significance and because of the potential risk of excessive bleeding in some individuals with intakes at higher levels, FDA concluded that the safety of menhaden oil was generally recognized only at levels that limit intake of EPA and DHA to 3.0 g/p/d.

FDA also concluded in the June 1997 final rule that 3.0 g/p/d of EPA and DHA is a safe level with respect to glycemic control (62 FR 30751 at 30753). This conclusion was based on FDA's review of a series of studies on non-insulin-dependent diabetics. Studies on type-II diabetics that reported increased glucose used higher amounts (4.5 to 8 g/p/d) of omega-3 fatty acids. One study found no change in fasting blood glucose levels among type-II (non-insulin-dependent) diabetics treated with 3.0 g/p/d EPA plus DHA for 2 weeks. Two other studies that used 3.0 g/p/d EPA plus DHA for 6 weeks and 2.7 g/p/d EPA plus DHA for 8 weeks found only transient increases in blood glucose halfway through their respective supplementation periods. Another study that used 3.0 g/p/d EPA plus DHA for 3 weeks found comparable increases in fasting blood glucose when either fish oil or safflower oil was fed, so the increase cannot be attributed specifically to omega-3 fatty acids. A study that compared the effects of fish oil and olive oil fed 3.0 g/p/d of EPA plus DHA did not find a difference in fasting glucose or glycosylated hemoglobin after fish oil supplementation compared to baseline; they did find a significant difference compared to the olive oil treatment, which produced changes in the opposite direction from fish oil. Based on its evaluation of the available information, FDA concluded in the June 1997 final rule that consumption of EPA and DHA in fish oils at 3.0 g/p/d by diabetics has no clinically significant effect on glycemic control, although higher amounts of EPA and DHA (4.5 g/p/d and above) remain of concern.

The June 1997 final rule also considered the reported effects of fish oil on LDL cholesterol levels in healthy persons with normal cholesterol levels, as well as in persons with diabetes mellitus, hypertension, abnormal blood lipid levels, and cardiovascular disease (62 FR 30751 at 30753 to 30754). As a result of its evaluation, FDA found that although reported study reports are variable, there appears to be a trend toward increased LDL cholesterol values with increased fish oil consumption in all population subgroups, with the magnitude of the increase appearing greater and more consistent in populations with abnormal blood lipid levels, hypertension, diabetes, and cardiovascular disease. Based on its evaluation, FDA concluded that 3.0 g/p/d of EPA and DHA is a safe level with respect to LDL cholesterol.

In the Federal Register of February 26, 2002 (67 FR 8744), FDA published a proposed rule to amend Sec. 184.1472 by reallocating the uses of menhaden oil in food, while maintaining the total daily intake of EPA and DHA from menhaden oil at a level not exceeding 3.0 g/p/d. The proposal was based on a citizen petition from the National Fish Meal and Oil Association. The maximum limit of 3.0 g/p/d on the total daily intake of EPA and DHA is a safeguard against the possible adverse effects discussed in the June 1997 final rule and the February 2002 proposed rule. The reallocation is performed by the following three actions: (1) Reducing the maximum levels of use of menhaden oil in some of the currently listed food categories; (2) adding additional food categories along with assigning maximum levels of use in these new categories; and (3) eliminating the listing of subcategories, e.g., cookies and crackers, breads and rolls, fruit pies and custard pies, and cakes, and including them under broader food categories, e.g., baked goods and baking mixes.

The purpose of the maximum use levels of menhaden oil in the food categories is to ensure that the total daily intake of EPA and DHA does not exceed 3.0 g/p/d (67 FR 8744 to 8745). When the June 1997 final rule published affirming that menhaden oil is GRAS for use as a direct human food ingredient with specific limitations, FDA considered food sources of EPA and DHA likely to be in the diet at that time, but the agency did not take into account that other sources of EPA and DHA might be developed in the future. The implicit basis for the restrictions in the menhaden oil regulation was that while menhaden oil might be blended with other oils to make a particular food product, the sum of DHA and EPA would not exceed 3.0 g/p/d because other oils were not significant sources of DHA and EPA. However, since publication of the proposed rule, FDA has received notices from three companies that have concluded that fish oils, other than menhaden oil, are GRAS for use in the same food categories as those currently listed in Sec. 184.1472(a)(3) at maximum use levels that are designed to assure that the combined daily intake of EPA and DHA would not exceed 3.0 g/p/d. These oils included small planktivorous pelagic fish body oil (oil derived primarily from sardine and anchovy fish) (Ref. 1), a fish oil concentrate (manufactured from oil extracted from edible marine fish species that normally include anchovy, sardine, jack mackerel, and mackerel) (Ref. 2), and tuna oil (Ref. 3). In each case, the company acknowledged the concerns raised by FDA in the June 1997 final rule and the proposed rule, about consumption of high levels of EPA and DHA.

Furthermore, in each case the company stated that its determination of GRAS status related only to the circumstance where its fish oil product is used as the sole added source of EPA and DHA in any given food category and is not combined or augmented with any other EPA/DHA-rich oil.

Because of developing interest in food ingredients that are sources of EPA and DHA, FDA now believes that it is necessary to state explicitly in the regulation that when menhaden oil is added as an ingredient in foods, it may not be used in combination with any other added oil that is a significant source of EPA and DHA. Without this restriction, the intake of DHA and EPA could exceed 3.0 g/p/d. Because this use restriction was not contained in the proposed rule, FDA is issuing this regulation as a tentative final rule under 21 CFR 10.40(f)(6). FDA will review any comments that are relevant to this condition of use and that are received within the 75-day comment period and will respond accordingly to these comments in the Federal Register.

FDA is also making an editorial update to Sec. 184.1472(a)(2)(iii) to reflect that the name for the Office of Premarket Approval has been changed to the Office of Food Additive Safety.

II. COMMENTS ON THE PROPOSED RULE

The agency provided 75 days for comments on the proposed rule. At the close of the comment period, the agency had received two comments that expressed concern regarding the environmental impact of the proposed rule. These two comments are addressed separately in section III of this document. The agency also received comments that were submitted from a fish oil company and a trade association that represents the fish oil industry that merely expressed general support for the agency's proposed rule. The other comments were from individual consumers who were opposed to the proposed rule.

Most of the comments FDA received expressing opposition to the proposed rule objected to declaring menhaden oil on food labels by the name "omega-3 fatty acids" or a variation of this name. Many of these comments asserted that "omega-3 fatty acids" is a misleading name for menhaden oil. Some comments were from vegetarians and vegans who stated that listing menhaden oil by the name "omega-3 fatty acids" will make it difficult for them to avoid this animal product in foods. There were also comments that stated that listing menhaden oil by the name "omega-3 fatty acids" will make it difficult for those with fish allergies to avoid this fish oil in foods.

The proposed rule did not address how menhaden oil is to be listed as an ingredient on food labels. Generally, under section 403(i)(2) of the Federal Food, Drug, and Cosmetic Act (21 U.S.C. 343(i)(2)), a food is misbranded unless its label bears the common or usual name of each ingredient. Although menhaden oil is a significant source of omega-3 fatty acids, FDA knows of no basis for considering omega-3 fatty acids to be its common or usual name. Any consideration of an alternative name for menhaden oil, such as "omega-3 fatty acids," is outside the scope of the proposed rule.

FDA also received comments from consumers asking the agency to consider the use of omega-3 fatty acids from sources other than menhaden fish, such as flax seed. FDA notes that although menhaden oil does contain omega-3 fatty acids (primarily EPA and DHA), omega-3 fatty acids are not the subject of the proposed rule. Therefore, the use of other oils is outside the scope of the proposed rule.

A few comments stated that the menhaden fish is unsuitable for human consumption and, therefore, oil from this fish should not be used as a food ingredient. As stated in the proposed rule, menhaden oil is already affirmed as generally recognized as safe as a direct human food ingredient (Sec. 184.1472). FDA has not received any new information or comments that would alter its previous determination that menhaden oil that meets the specifications in Sec. 184.1472 is generally recognized as safe for use in food under the conditions specified.

Some of the comments FDA received expressing opposition to the proposed rule were against the addition of menhaden oil to foods because of a concern about the possibility of high levels of contaminants in the menhaden oil due to bioaccumulation of these contaminants in the menhaden fish. Bioaccumulation describes the process that results in an increase in the concentration of a chemical in a biological organism over time, compared to the chemical's concentration in the environment. FDA has evaluated data on levels of various chemical contaminants, such as pesticides, polychlorinated biphenyls and dioxins in menhaden oil. Based on these data, FDA finds no basis for a safety concern from food uses of menhaden oil due to possible bioaccumulation of lipophilic chemical contaminants in the source fish.

III. Environmental Impact

The agency received two comments expressing concern about the impact that the proposed rule will have on the menhaden fish population. One comment asked whether this action will result in the "near extinction" of menhaden, mackerel, and sardines, and further asked how near extinction, if it results, would effect ocean ecosystems. The other comment asserted that menhaden are being overfished to extinction, and that because of their population decline, larger game fish populations off the Atlantic coast are dropping proportionately. Neither comment cited supporting data or information.

To ensure that the maximum sustainable yield of menhaden is not exceeded and to provide long-term production, the menhaden fisheries are monitored by the Atlantic and Gulf States Marine Fisheries Commissions (which are under the jurisdiction of the National Marine Fisheries Service (NMFS)), as well as by State authorities. If there is a threat to the long-term yield of a fishery, generally, limits will be imposed by these organizations. At present, the Atlantic and Gulf menhaden fisheries are considered to be healthy and not overfished. With regard to the impact that the proposed rule will have on mackerel and sardines, the United Nation's Foreign Agricultural Organization reports that the primary practice used to catch menhaden has one of the lowest discard ratios of any method for general commercial fishing. (Less than 3 percent by weight of the total menhaden catch are other species of fish.) In addition, NMFS reports a numerical bycatch incidence (i.e., fish that are unintentionally caught) of less than 0.1 percent for the menhaden fishing industry. For these reasons, the agency does not believe that the proposed rule would result in overfishing of menhaden or have a significant impact on other species of fish. In summary, the comments do not provide a basis on which to change the conclusions of the environmental analysis that was prepared for the proposed rule, as discussed in the following paragraph.

The agency has previously considered the environmental effects of affirming menhaden oil as GRAS as a direct human food ingredient, provided that the combined daily intake of EPA and DHA from menhaden oil does not exceed 3.0 g/p/d (62 FR 30751 at 30754). The analysis assumed that the maximum use levels would be completely used for each food category and concluded that this action will not have a significant impact on the menhaden population. This rule will reallocate the maximum levels among food categories but will not increase the total maximum allowable level. Therefore, our previous analysis is applicable. No new information or comments have been received that would affect the agency's previous determination that there is no significant impact on the human environment, and that an environmental impact statement is not required.

IV. ANALYSIS OF ECONOMIC IMPACTS

A. Final Regulatory Impact Analysis

FDA has examined the economic implications of this tentative final rule as required by Executive Order 12866. Executive Order 12866 directs agencies to assess all costs and benefits of available regulatory alternatives and, when regulation is necessary, to select regulatory approaches that maximize net benefits (including potential economic, environmental, public health and safety, and other advantages; distributive impacts; and equity). Executive Order 12866 classifies a rule as significant if it meets any one of a number of specified conditions, including: having an annual effect on the economy of $100 million, adversely affecting a sector of the economy in a material way, adversely affecting competition, or adversely affecting jobs. A regulation is also considered a significant regulatory action if it raises novel legal or policy issues. FDA has determined that this tentative final rule is not a significant regulatory action as defined by Executive Order 12866.

In the economic analysis of the proposed rule, we stated that the main benefit of this rule would be the expansion of the potential uses of menhaden oil made possible by the new maximum levels. Firms choosing to use menhaden oil will bear labeling and other costs. Because these costs are voluntary, they will be borne only if doing so is anticipated to be advantageous to the firm. Although firms making products that now use menhaden oil at levels below the current maximum but above the new maximum could bear potential compliance costs, we noted in the proposed rule that FDA did not know of any products in that category. We received no comments on this conclusion, or on any other part of the preliminary regulatory impact analysis.

B. Final Regulatory Flexibility Analysis

FDA has examined the economic implications of this tentative final rule as required by the Regulatory Flexibility Act (5 U.S.C. 601-612). If a rule has a significant economic impact on a substantial number of small entities, the Regulatory Flexibility Act requires agencies to analyze regulatory options that would lessen the economic effect of the rule on small entities. FDA finds that this tentative final rule would not have a significant economic impact on a substantial number of small entities.

The use of the menhaden oil by any small business is voluntary and will be undertaken only if doing so is anticipated to be advantageous to the small business. Small businesses would only bear a compliance cost if, as stated previously, they make products that are below the current maximum but above the new maximum.

The agency specifically requested comments from small businesses on its assumption that no small businesses make products that will be affected by reducing the maximum levels of menhaden oil in pies, cakes, fats, oils, fish products, and meat products. We received no comments on that assumption or any other part of the initial regulatory flexibility analysis.

C. Unfunded Mandates

Title II of the Unfunded Mandates Reform Act of 1995 (Public Law 104-4) requires cost-benefit and other analyses before any rulemaking if the rule would include a "Federal mandate that may result in the expenditure by State, local, and tribal governments, in the aggregate, or by the private sector, of $100,000,000 or more (adjusted annually for inflation) in any 1 year." The current inflation-adjusted statutory threshold is $112 million.

FDA has determined that this tentative final rule does not constitute a significant rule under the Unfunded Mandates Reform Act.

V. Paperwork Reduction Act

This tentative final rule contains no collections of information. Therefore, clearance by the Office of Management and Budget under the Paperwork Reduction Act of 1995 is not required.

VI. Federalism

FDA has analyzed this tentative final rule in accordance with the principles set forth in Executive Order 13132. FDA has determined that the tentative final rule does not contain policies that have substantial direct effects on the States, on the relationship between the National Government and the States, or on the distribution of power and responsibilities among the various levels of government. Because the agency concludes that this tentative final rule does not contain policies that have federalism implications as defined in the order, a federalism summary impact statement is not required.

VII. Comments

Interested person may submit to the Division of Dockets Management (see ADDRESSES) written or electronic comments regarding this document. Submit a single copy of electronic comments or two paper copies of any mailed comments, except that individuals may submit one paper copy. Comments are to be identified with the docket number found in the brackets in the heading of this document. Received comments may be seen in the Division of Dockets Management between 9 a.m. and 4 p.m., Monday through Friday.

VIII. REFERENCES

The following references have been placed on display in the Division of Dockets Management (see ADDRESSES) and may be seen by interested persons between 9 a.m. and 4 p.m., Monday through Friday.

[1]   GRAS notice GRN 000102, including the response letter to GRN 000102 dated September 3, 2002, from Alan M. Rulis of FDA to Edward Iorio of Jedwards International, available at *http://www. cfsan.fda.gov/ [tilde]rdb/opa-gras.html.*

[2]   GRAS notice GRN 000105, including the response letter to GRN 000105 dated October 15, 2002, from Alan M. Rulis of FDA to Nancy L. Schnell of Unilever United States, Inc., available at *http://www.cfsan.fda.gov/ [tilde]rdb/opa-gras.html.*

[3]   GRAS notice GRN 000109, including the response letter to GRN 000109 dated December 4, 2002, from Alan M. Rulis of FDA to Anthony Young of Piper Rudnick, LLP, available at *http://www.cfsan.fda.gov/[tilde]rdb/opa-gras.html.*

INDEX